I0415343

Enabled

ENABLED

OVERCOMING PARALYTIC POLIO

ELIZABETH HILLSTROM

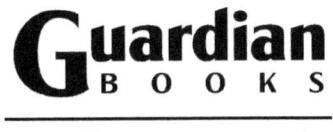

Belleville, Ontario, Canada

ENABLED

Copyright © 2017, Elizabeth Hillstrom

All Rights Reserved. No part of this publication may be reproduced, stored in a retrieval system or transmitted in any form or by any means—electronic, mechanical, photocopy, recording or any other— except for brief quotations in printed reviews, without the prior permission of the author.

Scripture taken from the HOLY BIBLE, NEW INTERNATIONAL VERSION ®. Copyright © 1973, 1978, 1984 by International Bible Society. Used by permission of Zondervan Publishing House. All rights reserved.

ISBN: 978-1-4600-0811-9
LSI Edition: 978-1-4600-0812-6
E-book ISBN: 978-1-4600-0813-3
(E-book available from the Kindle Store, KOBO and the iBooks Store)

Cataloguing data available from Library and Archives Canada

To order additional copies, visit:
www.essencebookstore.com

For more information, please contact:
Elizabeth Hillstrom
Hwheelers2@att.net

Guardian Books is an imprint of *Essence Publishing,* a Christian Book Publisher dedicated to furthering the work of Christ through the written word. For more information, contact:

20 Hanna Court, Belleville, Ontario, Canada K8P 5J2
Phone: 1-800-238-6376 • Fax: (613) 962-3055
Email: info@essence-publishing.com
Web site: www.essence-publishing.com

Guardian
B O O K S

Contents

L ife has often been described as a journey, rather like taking a very long vacation in which we travel from place to place enjoying the changing scenery, meeting different people, and delighting in new experiences. In some ways, life is like that, but in other important ways, it is not. In our journey through life, we do experience new places, people, and opportunities, but the agent that is driving much of this change is the passage of time rather than our own initiative and the critical changes are within ourselves rather than in our location.

Our lives on this earth seem like a journey because they are filled with changes. They also appear to be planned because they have a definite beginning and unfold in a consistent and predictable way from birth to old age. Plans presuppose the work of a planner, so following this line of reasoning brings up some crucial questions. Who or what made these plans for our lives and set them into motion? What are these plans, and what is the planner's purpose?

Long before we ever met, my husband, Kenneth, and I (Elizabeth) were both forced to wrestle with these questions because as young adults, our plans for ourselves were rudely interrupted by a viral disease known as paralytic poliomyelitis. After the acute infection passed, polio left both of us with serious physical disabilities. We had both performed well in high school and were highly motivated to get advanced training and enter some field of science. However, our disabilities made our plans to pursue higher education seem virtually impossible. Yet as we struggled to try to make sense of what had happened to us, to regain some physical strength and some understanding of what to do next, we discovered, independently, and in very different ways, that we were not alone on this very difficult stretch of the journey. The God of the Bible began to come alongside, and He changed the direction and circumstances of our lives in the most remarkable ways!

At one level, this book is an account of our journey through life—how God brought us together, enabled us to overcome formidable obstacles and achieve meaningful careers, and gave us a wonderful (and growing) family, an accessible home, and the resources and strength to manage all of this independently for most of our lives. At a much more profound and meaningful level, it is the story of how an awesome God led two ordinary people on an extraordinary journey to saving faith, to service, to deep purpose and meaning in life, and to an amazing (and eternal) relationship with Himself. My primary reason for writing our story is to share some of the many wonderful things that Ken and I learned firsthand about the Planner of all life journeys and the amazing love, provision, and future God offers to anyone who truly seeks a close, personal relationship with Him.

Chapter 1

Ken's Early Life

Ken was born in difficult times—in 1930, in the depths of the Great Depression. Elsie, Ken's mom, was the daughter of two Swedish immigrants, and Emil, his dad, had emigrated from Sweden to the United States with some friends just seven years earlier. These enterprising young men made their way to Chicago, taught themselves English, and learned carpentry and other trades with an daring but effective technique for acquiring on-the-job training. When they arrived in Chicago in the 1920s, construction jobs in the city were plentiful. They would hire onto a construction job, saying that they were carpenters, and learn all they could about the trade before their lack of skill became obvious and they were fired. Then, undaunted, they would simply move to a new job site several blocks away and apply the same tactics. After a few years (and many firings), they all became skilled tradesmen.

However, before Emil or his friends had opportunity to really prosper, the free-wheeling 1920s gave way to the desperate 1930s when jobs were very scare and most people had difficulty even earning enough to feed themselves. Ken retained many childhood memories of the tough times that his parents and their friends endured during that period. Emil could not find work for many months in those early years, so their only income was the fifteen dollars a week that Elsie was able to earn working at a pencil factory. This wasn't much, but given the severity of their situation, Ken's parents were very grateful for even that.

Since Elsie had the steady job, Emil stayed at home and took care of Ken for his first three years. Their times together generated some humorous incidents and a close bond between father and son, at least while Ken was young. One way Emil used to entertain Ken was by getting down on his hands and knees to play "horsie." Ken would then run to him and jump on his back for a wild noisy ride. After one particularly vigorous romp, Emil started to get up, felt a very sharp pain in his back, and discovered that he was stuck! He could not change his position in any way without severe pain. And he remained stuck on his hands and knees for about twenty minutes. Ken was delighted because it appeared that Emil was ready to roughhouse some more. Emil could not raise an arm to fend Ken off without pain, but neither did he dare let Ken jump on his back. Nor were his commands to stop very effective. Ken didn't take him seriously because, in spite of his pain, Emil could not stop laughing at Ken's antics.

When he was a little older, Ken recalls, city employees periodically delivered "County Boxes" of free food to his parents' apartment (and to those of their neighbors) to help families survive. Ken's parents were not alone in their need because many people depended upon these boxes and other free food to supplement their diets. They simply did not have enough money to buy the food they needed. During this very difficult part of the Depression, young, unmarried men without jobs who were living away from their families were in even greater need. They did not qualify for County Boxes, which were reserved for families, and they usually could not even afford a place to live. They could get one meal a day by standing in long lines at soup kitchens, which were set up to distribute free food to those who were particularly destitute.

One of Emil's friends, Carl, found himself in this predicament. Since Carl was homeless, Emil invited him to come to their apartment every night so he could at least sleep on their sofa in the living room. To his parents' amusement and embarrassment, Ken, then about two, started calling this young man "Sofa" when he saw him because he had heard that word so often when Carl was there.

Ken also described early memories of garbage and ice wagons pulled along by horses in the city streets. Vendors sold the ice in big chunks so their customers could place these blocks of ice in "ice boxes" to keep food cool. Ken and other kids liked to chase after the ice wagons, hoping that the driver would notice them and throw them some ice chips to eat. For obvious reasons, the garbage wagons held no such attraction!

As a boy, Ken lived with his parents on the third floor of a brick, three-flat apartment building on the north side of Chicago. It was within reasonable walking distance to Wrigley Field, so Ken and his friends would walk or bike there while a baseball game was in session and wait at the gates. During the seventh inning, the proprietors would open the gates, inviting anyone who was waiting to come in and watch the rest of the game without charge. Sometimes while waiting, the boys would position themselves behind the wall around the outfield and watch for baseballs that were hit out of the park. They would scoop these up and take them home as souvenirs.

Ken loved biking, running, and other athletic activities. He developed very strong legs, and according to his boyhood friends, he was a fast sprinter and an agile football player. As teenagers, this group would ride their bikes to Lake Michigan beaches to swim and to the parks along Lake Michigan to play ball. When they had the good fortune of having a little money, they visited Riverview Amusement Park.

The Depression wore on through all the 1930s, but Ken's family and their neighbors learned to get by on less and continued to cope. As government job programs were put in place, the employment problem eased a bit. However, it didn't fully abate until the coming of World War II in 1941, which created enormous demands for tanks, planes, weapons, food, and other supplies. These new demands provided abundant work for both men and women. By this time, Emil was beyond the prime age for enlisting, but he found plenty of work as a skilled carpenter; in particular, helping to build barracks and other buildings at the Great Lakes Naval Training Station on Lake Michigan.

Ken attended several city schools while growing up. In grade school and junior high, by his own admission, he was an indifferent student at best, merely skimming by, doing as little work as possible, and barely making passing grades. This frustrated Ken's parents and teachers because they were sure he could do much better. Ken, however, was simply dedicated to enjoying life and having fun, not anticipating how this would impact his future.

In spite of his lackluster performance at school, Ken actually learned to read early and quickly and enjoyed reading things at home that piqued his interest. When the ominous events of World War II began to unfold in Europe in the early 1940s, as Ken was approaching his twelfth birthday, he began to realize that these events could threaten his life and the lives of everyone around him. He felt a great need to try to understand what was happening in the world and became strongly motivated to learn as much as he could about world events. His search for information aroused his interest in current events, geography, economics, and world history, as well as the events in World War II. These interests grew deeper and remained with him for the rest of his life.

Ken began reading newspapers, magazines, and books on these topics, listened avidly to news reports on radio, and eagerly went to the local theater with Elsie every weekend to see the latest newsreels on the war. He also obtained maps so he could see where battles were occurring and used them to plot various developments and troop movements. It was at about this time that he also evidenced a rather surprising but genuine interest in farming! Elsie was really taken aback one day when Ken asked her if he could subscribe to the *Farm Journal*. However, she followed her instincts and gave him the money for the subscription. (Incidentally, Ken continued to get that magazine for a number of years, even renewing it for a time after we were married.)

Ken fully committed his life to Jesus when he was fourteen years old. Many factors led him to this decision. For one, although he had grown up with an unbelieving father, he had been nurtured by a believing mother and a strong church family from the time he was four. Elsie had been raised in the church; however, as a young adult she had slipped away from her faith. It was during this time that she met and married Emil, who was not a believer. After Ken was born, Elsie had a change of heart, recommitted her life, and started attending Immanuel Mission Covenant Church in Chicago.

Emil was raised in a strong Christian family in Sweden but left that country with undeserved bitterness towards his father and the Christianity his father embraced. Early in his marriage, Emil would sometimes attend church functions with Elsie, but he never committed his own life to Jesus. His stated reason for not doing so was both frank and unsettling: "I know there is a God and that He has rules, but I am going to live my life my own way." Although Emil eventually stopped going to church, to his credit he did not directly interfere with Elsie's or Ken's involvement. Still, the marked differences between Emil's beliefs and those of Elsie and Ken became an increasing source of strife and grief as their interests, beliefs, and values continued to diverge.

Elsie enrolled Ken in the Cradle Roll at Immanuel when he was four, and he grew up attending church at least three times a week. The pastor spoke clearly and often about Heaven, Hell, and the need for everyone to repent and accept Jesus Christ as Lord. As Ken matured, he was involved in youth programs and camp activities associated with the church. In addition, most of the church members at Immanuel were Swedish immigrants or the children of Swedish immigrants, and many of these members knew each other or other members of their families before coming to America. The friendships and ties between these families were deep, and they would frequently visit with each other at their respective homes. Not surprisingly, Ken's best friends in his preteen and teenage years were other young men from this church.

Another important factor that motivated Ken to surrender his life to the Lord was the onset of World War II and the increasing manifestations of that war all around him. In junior high and high school, Ken had to take public transportation to get to school. During that time, there were increasing numbers of soldiers, marines, and sailors in uniform all over Chicago, and he would see them everywhere. Often he would find himself sitting close to them in the street cars. As he studied these men in uniform at close range, it dawned on him that many were very young—some only five years older than he. He also began to realize that with the impending invasion of Europe, many of these same young men would lose their lives. With the impeccable logic that would mark his entire adult life, it suddenly became very clear to him that he, also, could die young. This realization shook him deeply. Death was suddenly a very real possibility, and he was not saved! It was on D-Day, June 6, 1944, at the very beginning of the Allies' massive invasion of Europe, that Ken fully accepted Jesus as his own personal Savior and Lord.

This turning point brought Ken a sense of peace but also marked the onset of new challenges. Ken quickly recognized that accepting Jesus as Savior and Lord was just the first step to a very different kind of life. He now had to "walk the talk," grow up, and live up to his responsibilities. He needed to live in obedience to the Bible and to start working hard in school to become a responsible adult and an effective Christian. He also realized that this was not going to be easy. He needed to overcome poor study habits, to learn what he had failed to learn in grade school and in junior high, and to do this as quickly as possible. His increased awareness of his past failures and their consequences plus his emerging sense of responsibility brought with them increasing fears that he would not be able to measure up or, worse yet, that his life would be a failure.

Ken's freshman year at Amundsen High School in Chicago was fraught with struggle. In spite of intense efforts on his part, his grades inched up only slowly. To make matters worse, in the middle of that school year, Emil began drinking heavily and staying out late at night. Then he decided to leave Elsie and Ken and live with another woman he had met. A few months later Emil returned, telling Elsie he was sorry and asking her permission to move back. This she granted, but their relationship was never the same. Understandably, Emil's behavior and the pain it inflicted upon both Ken and Elsie upset Ken very deeply. It also added to Ken's own fears and insecurities as he began to realize that he might have to be responsible not only for providing for himself but for his mother as well.

Emil's actions also exacerbated the ongoing shame that Ken and Elsie experienced in the presence of their friends at church because their families were intact and their marriages seemed good and stable. For a long time, Ken had felt like a second-class member at his church because his dad was always missing. But now, after Emil's unfaithfulness, Ken felt deeply ashamed. Although neither Ken nor Elsie experienced any negative or condemning comments from their long-time friends at church, both became uncomfortable there. They started attending other, larger evangelical churches where their family situation was not known and was not as likely to become such an issue.

One salutary effect that all this trouble produced in both Ken and Elsie was a growing dependence upon the Lord alone for strength and sustenance and a growing assurance that He was right there by their side. As different crises came up during this period, Elsie began to get tangible "feelings of assurance" from the Lord. This was a sense that everything would resolve in a good way, according to God's will—in answer to her specific prayers. Ken (and later I) would come to treasure those assurances. On Ken's part, the Lord used those difficult times to strengthen his determination to keep on keeping on, no matter what. With the Lord's help, he was not going to give up or give in, and he refused to capitulate to his strong bouts of fear. Through sheer determination, effort, and prayer, he redoubled his efforts at school and slowly raised his grades.

At the end of that first year at Amundsen High School, encouraged by his academic progress there, Ken decided to take on an even greater challenge. He transferred from Amundsen to Lane Technical High School, a large school with high admission standards. At that time, it admitted only men. Its emphasis was on preparing students who were seeking rigorous training in engineering and science. In his three years at Lane, Ken enjoyed playing football and concentrated on learning and honing his study skills. When he graduated from Lane in 1948, he had maintained a 95.2 grade-point average over all three years and was awarded a certificate of honor for his academic excellence.

When Ken transferred to Lane, he was thinking about engineering as a career but later decided that medicine would be more to his liking. Toward that end, in his senior year at Lane, he applied for the premedical programs at both Northwestern University in Chicago and Wheaton College in Wheaton, Illinois. Ken's strong preference was to attend Wheaton College because of its Christian environment, its strong premedical program, and the possibility of playing football there. However, in spite of his very strong academic credentials, he was not accepted at Wheaton that first year. In 1948, when Ken first applied, there were large numbers of veterans of World War II who were also seeking to enter college under the GI Bill of Rights. At that time, Wheaton College was giving preference to qualified returning veterans. Ken was accepted at Northwestern University, so he attended there as a freshman, meanwhile putting in an application to transfer to Wheaton College for the 1949-1950 school year. This time his application to Wheaton was accepted.

Ken went to Wheaton College early that fall so he could attend Wheaton's preseason football camp, which was held on a lakeside property in Wisconsin. Since Ken really enjoyed this sport and was very good at it, he participated enthusiastically in the training. That year, the late-summer weather was quite warm and all the team members would get very hot and sweaty during practice. The gentle beach and cool lake water nearby proved irresistible, and Ken and some of the other team members would often take a quick dip in the lake to cool off after practice.

This activity seemed harmless enough at the time, but it was probably the cause of a series of events that would soon change Ken's life dramatically. Camp ended, and all seemed well. Ken started classes on campus, but after only three days, he became very ill. His temperature soared, and he had very severe headaches along with serious muscle pain and weakness. In the college infirmary, the attending physician quickly identified the probable cause. Ken had all the signs of a disease that was widespread and greatly feared in 1949—paralytic poliomyelitis.

Poliomyelitis, also known as "infantile paralysis" or "polio," is caused by a virus that flourishes in lakes and streams. At that time, polio epidemics were common in the United States and other developed countries, especially in late summer and early fall. At the peak of these epidemics, thousands of people, the great majority of them children, would fall ill every year. Polio was a terrifying disease, not only because it could cause death or permanent physical disability, but also because there were no effective medicines or procedures that could be used to combat the infection once it gained a foothold. One could only hope and pray that the victim's immune system could get the upper hand before the damage became too severe. Fortunately, when the Salk and Sabin vaccines became available in the early 1950s and as larger and larger percentages of the population in this country were vaccinated, new infections were virtually eliminated. They were rare by 1959.

The effects of polio varied greatly depending upon which of the three types of virus was present, the age of the victim, and the effectiveness of the victim's immune response. The most common type caused mild, flu-like symptoms and then disappeared. Many infected by this type of polio never even realized it. A second form, bulbar polio, was deadly, but fortunately, it was also rare. It would rapidly destroy neurons in the spinal cord and lower part of the brain that controlled the muscles necessary for breathing.

Paralytic polio was fairly common and could also greatly impair breathing, but it generally targeted neurons in the spinal cord that controlled voluntary movement. Its effects varied a great deal. It might cause paralysis or weakness of an arm, a leg, both legs or arms, trunk muscles, or any combination of these, depending upon which parts of the spinal cord it attacked. The destructive phase of polio usually passed in a week or so, and some recovery was possible for up to a year or more. However, in most cases, victims were left with permanent paralysis. In addition, paralytic polio often produced more severe effects in young adults than it did in children.

Very soon after the doctor saw Ken at the college infirmary, he was transferred by ambulance to what was then the Municipal Contagious Disease Hospital in Chicago where he was placed in a confining, whole-body respirator known as the "iron lung." These machines were large, heavy-duty, metal tubes on wheels that were made especially for polio patients who had developed serious breathing problems. They encased the entire body, except for the patient's neck and head, and greatly restricted movement. To relieve possible feelings of claustrophobia and to enable patients to see more than just the ceiling, they also had small, adjustable mirrors positioned just above the patient's head that could be angled so patients could at least see some of what was around or behind them.

The doctors placed Ken in an iron lung as a precautionary measure because at this early stage of the infection, they could not know whether or to what extent Ken's breathing might become impaired.

The hospital, because it was built to treat contagious diseases, had large numbers of small cubicles in which individual patients could be isolated. Visitors could look into the cubicles through windows and see the patient they were visiting and perhaps wave or mouth a few words from outside, but no physical contact with the patient was permitted except by doctors and trained nurses. For Ken, the added restriction of being immobilized in an iron lung made any meaningful communication very difficult, and this added greatly to his fears and feelings of isolation.

Ken was in Municipal Contagious Disease Hospital for twelve days. During the first few days, his fever raged and he remained confined in the big machine in the small cubicle. During this time, he discovered that he could no longer move his legs. Ken, who had always delighted in vigorous physical activity, was overwhelmed by this loss. He also began to struggle with intense fears of what might lie in his future. Would he be able to recover movement? Would he still be physically capable of becoming a medical doctor, as he had hoped? Would he even be able to walk again? Worse yet, would he be too disabled to do anything meaningful with his life? In the midst of all this turbulence, he tried to pray, but fierce waves of fear, uncertainty, and loss seemed to swamp his most determined efforts.

Another circumstance that added greatly to Ken's distress was his awareness of what was happening all around him. Although he couldn't move or see very much, he could still hear the heart-wrenching dramas that were unfolding in nearby cubicles. He would periodically hear the sounds and words of doctors and nurses dealing with various emergencies, and he also heard the cries of utter despair and grief as three different families watched their stricken children die from polio. All this was incredibly distressing, and it sent Ken very close to his breaking point. After the third child died, Ken was overwhelmed with both grief and anger. In desperation and protest, he cried out loud to God that this was about as close to Hell as anyone could get!

It was at that moment, while half expecting a reprimand from God for his outburst, that Ken was suddenly and inexplicably filled "with a most beautiful sense of peace and joy." While he was still marveling at this dramatic turn of events, in his mind he very clearly heard the Lord tell him that he would live! Moreover, his life would be very meaningful! This assurance was an enormous comfort. Ken suddenly understood that God was right there with him, continuing to guide his life. God still loved him. And God still had a plan and a purpose for his life. In the lingering peace, joy, and assurance of that encounter, Ken let go of his fears and fell into a deep and restful sleep.

He was awakened rather abruptly the next morning by unfamiliar voices. Several doctors and nurses were beside him, smiling and assuring him that he had passed the crisis. The fever had passed, and Ken was breathing normally, so he was removed from the iron lung and transferred to a regular room where he could visit with family and friends and begin living a much more normal life. With deep thankfulness for his life and with the reassurance he had received from the Lord, Ken began his very long and arduous journey to recovery. On September 30, 1949, Ken was transferred to Grant Hospital in Chicago where he would remain for another nine months before he could finally leave for home.

Fighting Back

U pon his arrival at Grant Hospital, Ken's doctors immediately evaluated his physical status. Although polio
had apparently spared his respiratory system, it had
caused extensive paralysis in the lower half of his body. The only
muscle Ken could move in either leg was a small one in a big toe.
His leg muscles, once so strong and prominent, were shrinking
rapidly. In addition, many of Ken's back and abdominal muscles
were paralyzed or considerably weakened. Only his arms, shoulders, upper back, and neck muscles remained unaffected.

As Ken struggled to come to terms with these dramatic losses
and what they might mean for his future, he questioned his doctors intently. Did they think he would be able to walk again? Did
they think he would be able to attend college? Would it still possible for him to pursue a career in medicine? The doctors could not
answer these questions definitively at this early stage of his recovery,
however they were pretty sure he would not be able to walk normally (or any other way, for that matter) and they were doubtful
that he could regain the strength he would need to attend college.

This information could have been devastating, but Ken remembered the powerful encouragement he had received from the Lord
and refused to let his fears and emotions get the upper hand. He was
realistic about his situation, but he also reasoned that since the Lord
had promised that he would have a very meaningful life, this must

mean that he would have meaningful work to do. Moreover, if there was work to do, the Lord would surely give him the strength and capabilities he would need to carry it out. Ken did not expect a miraculous healing but believed, rather, that if he trusted the Lord and worked hard to do all that he could do to recover and to get an education, God would supply whatever else he needed.

Ken's optimism and quiet confidence in this situation had an impact upon everyone around him. Friends, family, and those who came to know him at the hospital could not help but ask how he could have such peace and confidence. And when they asked, Ken would gladly tell them about his amazing encounter with the Lord. Word of Ken's testimony spread among several churches in Chicago, even reaching a young radio announcer, Bill Pierce, who was then working for Moody Radio. Bill asked Ken for a radio interview and brought the necessary equipment right into the hospital. Through this broadcast, Ken was able to share his testimony with many more people.

When I heard this account years later, I too asked Ken how he was able to remain so calm and assured in the hospital in the face of so much loss. Ken told me that main reason was the absolute clarity and reality of his encounter with the Lord. He also explained that much of the inner turmoil he experienced at the hospital had actually been with him months *before* polio struck! His battle with polio had merely intensified these underlying fears and concerns. The basic issues that were troubling him were doubts about God and the reality of his faith, plus his deep-seated fears of failure and of not measuring up as a Christian. Ken's dramatic encounter with God answered these fundamental questions. It convinced him that God was real and that His promises of forgiveness and of salvation were true. It confirmed to him that God did love him and that human life did indeed have meaning and purpose. It also reassured him that God had a plan for his life, even if that plan might be very different from the plan he had mapped out for himself.

Chapter 2: Fighting Back

Ken worked diligently in therapy and slowly began building strength in normal and newly weakened muscles. Since his arms, shoulders, hands, and upper back were strong, he learned to use a manual wheelchair and to make transfers to and from it to the bed, regular chairs, etc. fairly quickly. The loss of thirty pounds, mostly from muscle atrophy, made transferring less difficult. However, learning to "walk" again would prove to be much more difficult!

Even though none of the muscles in Ken's legs were showing any signs of recovery, Ken's orthopedic doctor did want to see if he might be able to learn to walk with the aid of crutches and long leg braces (which extended from mid-thigh to the bottom of each foot and could be locked straight to prevent his knees from buckling). He was also concerned about the weaknesses in Ken's back and abdominal muscles and didn't know if these were strong enough to hold Ken upright while he was standing with the leg braces. He had also discovered some curvature in Ken's spine and was concerned that having him stand upright might make that worse. To be safe, he ordered a sturdy brace for Ken's back and torso that extended from his arm pits to his hips.

As you can probably imagine, when Ken first saw (and lifted) the new braces for the first time, he despaired of ever being able to use these to walk in any meaningful way. At that time, braces were very heavy and cumbersome because they were constructed of iron or steel and leather. Ken quickly realized that even learning how to put these braces on without help would be a challenge. His first therapy session with the braces bore that out. He had to have assistance putting on all three braces and then needed two people to lift him up on his feet. Then, once he was on his feet, he couldn't even stay upright without help. In the next session, he learned to steady himself by holding on to some bars with his hands. However, even with a lot more time and exercise, he wasn't even close to being able to walk with crutches and braces.

After nine months of recovery and therapy at Grant Hospital, Ken was managing well with the wheelchair and was able to transfer to and from the bed, other chairs and even the floor just using his arms, so his doctors decided that it was time for him to leave for home. However, that prospect presented a whole new set of difficulties. Home was a third-floor apartment in a three-flat apartment building in Chicago. The only access to the apartment was via two long sets of stairs. Those stairs did have sturdy handrails of both sides, but at that point they still created an impossible barrier. When Ken was finally released from Grant Hospital on June 25, 1950, he had just passed his twentieth birthday. He had to be carried up to the apartment on a stretcher and didn't know if he would ever be able to leave and re-enter that space on his own power.

Ken felt very ambivalent that day. He was grateful to be going home, but he also struggled mightily with fears of being confined to his parents' small apartment for months or even years at a time. He also dreaded the prospect of being caught in the middle of the heated arguments between his parents with no way to escape. Ken recognized that his anxieties were getting out of hand, so he forced himself to stop and remember the Lord's promises. This enabled him to push his fears aside and focus on two essential goals. He was determined to do everything in his power to learn to walk and to complete his education. Without these two achievements, he could not hope to eventually live on his own.

While he was in Grant Hospital, Ken had plenty of opportunity to talk with doctors and interns and to consider whether he should still pursue a career in medicine. Slowly and rather painfully, he realized that this wasn't really feasible—he needed to find a vocation that was not so physically demanding. In spite of Ken's dislike of and struggles with math courses in school, he did have a strong interest in statistics and in working with numbers, so he decided to seek training as an accountant or an actuary. He also discovered that he could take some of the college-level courses he would need for this kind of training at home, through correspondence courses from the University of Illinois at Champaign-Urbana. So he signed up for a couple of courses soon after coming home from the hospital and went right to work on them.

Mathematics courses taken by correspondence could be challenging because feedback from the instructors was necessarily limited. Students were pretty much on their own to figure out what the text was teaching. For each lesson, Ken was required to complete a large number of problems and send these in to be graded. Texts gave the answers to some problems, but it was still up to the student to write out all of the steps to each solution. After completing all the lessons, Ken would take a proctored, two-hour exam covering the entire course. Ninety percent or more of his grade was based on that test. Taking courses this way was very time consuming and somewhat risky as far as grades were concerned, but they did provide a way for Ken to advance his education from the apartment while continuing to build his physical strength. As Ken tackled increasingly advanced math courses this way, he discovered that he enjoyed the challenge and was able to do the work exceptionally well.

Before Ken left Grant Hospital, his doctor and family worked out a plan for his continued rehabilitation at home. Elsie and Emil assisted him with daily exercises, and Miss Hill, a visiting nurse, made weekly visits to observe and supervise. Ken and his parents also devised additional ways to rebuild his strength. Emil created a chin-up bar that could be placed in a doorway for exercise and then easily removed. Later, he also built a set of three steps with sturdy handrails, very similar to the stairs leading up to the apartment.

Ken was determined to learn to walk using his braces and crutches, but he was sure that the heavy back brace was making this impossible. His orthopedic doctor, Ferdinand Seidler, had warned him that the curvature in his spine might get worse without the back brace, and if this happened, he would need back surgery and have to spend months in a heavy body cast until it healed. Nevertheless, Ken took a calculated risk and stopped using that brace except when Miss Hill was present. After making that decision, Ken began regaining strength in his back and abdomen fairly rapidly.

Miss Hill noticed these changes and finally asked Ken if he was still using his back brace every day. He admitted that he was not and told her his reasons. At first she was hesitant, but eventually she went along with Ken's strategy because she could see for herself the obvious improvements in his strength. As time went by, she even became a valued co-conspirator, working with him to find new exercises and innovative techniques that would help him reach his goals.

After several months had passed, Ken scheduled a follow-up appointment with Dr. Seidler. He had asked Ken to get new X-rays of his back and to bring these along because he was sure Ken would need corrective back surgery. At the appointment, the doctor set up Ken's X-rays and studied them closely. As he did, he first looked puzzled, then startled, and finally, for a long time, he just stared in disbelief. Ken's spine was normal! The exercise had successfully strengthened his back and abdominal muscles, and the curvature had disappeared. To Ken's and Elsie's absolute delight, in his heavy, expressive German accent, Dr. Seidler finally conceded, "So-o-o-o! It is gone!" There was nothing more he could do but to give Ken his heart-felt congratulations and encouragement to continue what he had been doing.

Before Ken could learn to walk independently with his crutches and braces, he had to learn how to get up to a standing position by himself. This required several tricky maneuvers that always posed some risk of falling. After putting on his leg braces in bed and transferring to his wheelchair, Ken would position his crutches against an empty space on a wall, back his chair against the wall beside them, and lock his wheelchair brakes. He then straightened his legs out in front of him and locked the leg braces. Next he pulled his right leg across the left leg and turned the upper half of his body in the same direction, using his arms and the wheelchair armrests to pivot his body 180 degrees. At this point, his legs were parallel and the front of his body faced the chair and the floor. He then lifted his upper body with both arms and used his hip muscles to pull his straightened legs up under him. He next reached up to the wall, maneuvering himself into a vertical position with his hands and arms. Finally he balanced himself carefully with one hand on the wall, using the other hand to retrieve his crutches and slip them under his arms.

As Ken continued building his upper body strength, he also gained better balance. He couldn't actually take steps, one leg at a time, because the muscles that would allow him to do that were paralyzed. However, he did have enough hip strength to swing his entire lower body forward. To take a "step," Ken would balance himself on the braces, lift both crutches and move them forward about a step, shift his weight to the crutches, lift and swing his body forward, and again regain his balance. This method was slow and very risky at first because it required close concentration, a lot of arm and shoulder strength, and a very good sense of balance. However, with time and practice, Ken became quite proficient at walking in this manner.

While he was learning to walk, Ken and Miss Hill also worked on a strategy for conquering the stairs. This was undoubtedly the toughest challenge of all because Ken couldn't bend his knees with the braces and had to rely entirely upon his upper body strength for lift and for balance. He probably would have failed in this endeavor without the three-step structure that Emil had built for him to use for practice. With it, Ken could try different strategies and maneuvers with minimal risk. If he slipped and fell, at least he wouldn't fall very far. It would have been far too dangerous for him to try to learn on the steps leading down from the apartment.

With time and a lot of effort, Ken learned to go up steps by holding onto the left handrail with both hands, using hip muscles on his right side to swing his right leg up onto the next step, using his arms to pull his body up, and finally using hip muscles to bring the left leg up on the step. He would descend the steps backward, letting one leg drop to the lower step, shifting his weight to that leg, and then positioning himself with his arms so he could swing the other leg down. After repeating these maneuvers successfully many times on the practice steps, he was finally ready to tackle the real stairs outside the apartment door.

At first he only attempted going down to the first landing and back up, because doing only this required a lot of effort. Later he made it to the second floor and back. Finally, in the latter part of May 1951, shortly after his twenty-first birthday and eleven months after being transported up those steps on a stretcher, Ken made it down to the first floor. He went outside the front door with a wonderful new sense of freedom and thanksgiving to the Lord and then successfully climbed all the way back up to the apartment. He was elated with this achievement. Because he had persevered, kept taking the necessary risks, and kept trusting the Lord, he had seen one impossible obstacle after another fall away. This gave him a renewed sense of confidence that the Lord would help him reach his other goals.

By the time I met Ken, he had been climbing those stairs almost daily for several years. When I first accompanied him up the stairs, I was amazed. The process was somewhat slow, but he did it so smoothly that I failed to appreciate what an incredible accomplishment it actually was.

After Ken was able to get up and down the stairs without tiring, he started training to build up his endurance while walking. He realized that he needed to be much stronger to face the rigors of living on campus and getting to classes on time. His first goal was to get down the steps, immediately walk one-fourth of a city block and back, and then ascend the stairs. After that, he lengthened the walk to two, three, and then four city blocks. Elsie would walk with him, timing him to see how long these trips took. Time was important

because Ken knew that on campus he might have only fifteen minutes to get from one class to another. After Ken could comfortably
walk four blocks, he started strapping books to his crutches on these
trips to increase his endurance. Once he could do the stairs and
immediately walk four blocks with the books without stopping to
rest, he was ready to try taking classes on campus again.

Ken realized that functioning on campus would require additional skills with his crutches and braces because his wheelchair
would be useless there. There were no ramps into buildings, no elevators inside, and no curb cuts at street crossings. He would have
to learn to get up and down curbs (with nothing stationary to hold
on to) and in and out of the specialized writing-arm chairs in the
classrooms while using only the crutches and braces.

To minimize the number of new challenges he would face on
campus, Ken started with two summer-school classes. That way
Emil could provide daily transportation and Ken wouldn't have to
struggle with inaccessible housing or with ice and snow on walks
and steps in winter weather. By the end of that summer of 1952,
with the Lord's unfailing provision, Ken passed another milestone.
He had overcome the curb and the chair challenges and earned A's
in both of his courses. Armed with these successes, he applied for
full-time status for the fall of 1953. While he was waiting, he completed more correspondence courses and attended summer school
again right before fall classes started.

Wheaton College did admit Ken as a full-time student that fall
but not without some reservations. Those who made the decision
simply didn't know of anyone with significant physical disabilities
who had made it through college, so they had legitimate doubts,
especially about how Ken would withstand the rigors of living on
campus, getting to classes, and really being able to take advantage
of the training he was seeking. Still, the dean and others on the
admissions committee felt they needed to give him a chance, especially since he had been a full-time student at Wheaton when he

had come down with polio and he did have excellent academic credentials. So even though no one said anything to suggest it, Ken sensed that he was on some kind of informal probation and concluded that he had to prove not only that he could do the work but that he could also excel at it.

For the fall semester, Ken deliberately scheduled all of his classes on Tuesdays and Thursdays because he knew that he could not get into the college dining hall. With that schedule, he could eat a large breakfast at home on Tuesday mornings before Emil drove him to his first class. He would have his next full meal at home on Thursday evening after Emil picked him up. In between times, he ate only what he was able to bring with him from home. On Tuesday and Wednesday nights, Ken stayed in a house located about two blocks from Blanchard Hall, where most of his classes were located. Like many houses of the time, it had several front steps, narrow doorways, and small bathrooms, so Ken had to manage there without his wheelchair as well.

His first six weeks back in residence were difficult. Just getting to his first class was tiring. He had to maneuver down the front steps of the house, walk about two blocks up a fairly steep hill, navigate two curbs, and then climb a long flight of stairs in Blanchard Hall to get there. In addition to the physical challenges, Ken felt great pressure to excel in all of his classes to prove that he could succeed on campus. He literally spent all the time he had available studying.

One of the classes Ken was most concerned about that first semester was Integral Calculus. The math courses he had taken by correspondence had prepared him well, but he didn't have as much time to study for it as he would have liked. While doing correspondence, he could take fewer courses and study at his own pace. At Wheaton, for financial reasons, Ken was carrying a full course load and had much less time to prepare for each class. To make matters worse, these courses were all set up to have six-week exams during the same week. The pressure he felt that week was intense!

The calculus test was his first exam, and Ken believed that his performance on that test would enable him to assess whether or not he was going to be able to succeed in residence or not. It seemed to him that all he had been working toward so diligently the last four years was now on the line. Doing well on this test would confirm that he was truly in the Lord's will. If he did poorly, he wasn't even sure he could stay in school. With all these concerns weighing on his mind, Ken prepared for this and his other six-week tests as well as he possibly could. He prayed earnestly for peace and assurance, but he still felt very anxious.

When Ken received the calculus test, he read the first problem and nearly panicked because he couldn't remember how to do it. He read the second problem and couldn't remember how to do that one either. He bowed his head and breathed a desperate prayer to the Lord for help and felt some peace. He glanced quickly at the third problem and was reassured when he recognized the solution. He then successfully worked his way through the remaining problems and finally went back to the first and second, completing those as well. He finished on time but had little opportunity to review his work. Just as he was finishing, he saw a drop of blood spatter on the chair arm right next to his exam. Under all the pressure, his nose had started to bleed!

Even though the calculus exam was challenging, Ken later discovered that he had made a perfect score on it. Not only that, but he had scored very highly on all his other six-week exams as well. He was elated. The Lord was still with him and was guiding his steps. He knew then that no matter what new challenges he would face, by working hard and trusting the Lord day by day, he could complete his bachelor's degree.

The dean and others who had been concerned about Ken's ability to succeed on campus also took note of his six-week grades and quickly decided to do whatever they could to help him complete his work, including moving all of his classes to the first floor of Blanchard Hall. This helped immensely. However, Ken still didn't know whether he could even walk to Blanchard when there was snow or ice coating the walkway. Yet day by day, every Tuesday and Thursday throughout the entire winter, there was always a way! Professors who knew about Ken's situation and even the dean would drop by to take him up the hill to Blanchard in their own cars when it was unusually cold or sidewalks and steps were treacherous.

Ken continued as a full-time student at Wheaton College until he finished his bachelor's degree, with a major in mathematics and a minor in English literature. He graduated, *magna cum laude*, in the spring of 1955 and then went on to complete a master's degree in applied mathematics at Northwestern University in June of 1957. In the fall of 1957, with the Lord's obvious leading, he began what would become a thirty-two-year career at Argonne National Laboratory. Ken did not become an accountant or an actuary like he thought he might, but instead he found himself on the ground floor of a career that he hadn't even heard of—the newly emerging discipline of computer science. He worked in the Department of Applied Mathematics and Computer Science, where he did research and developed software for scientific experiments that other researchers at Argonne were carrying out.

Ken found this work both challenging and gratifying, but for reasons that were not clear to him at that time, after a couple of years at Argonne, he began to feel very restless. While he was praying about the issue and trying to identify the reasons for his restlessness, it came to his mind that perhaps what he needed to do was to get further training. Therefore, in the fall of 1960, he took temporary leave from Argonne and drove downstate to the University of Illinois, at Champaign-Urbana, to begin coursework for a PhD in mathematics. Little did he realize that this move was part of a greater plan that would eventually bring him the added meaning and fulfillment that the Lord had promised.

Chapter 3

Betty's Early Life

L ike Ken, I (Elizabeth or "Betty") was born in a time of trouble and in Illinois, but in a farmhouse midway down the state rather than in Chicago. The year was 1941, only months before the United States officially entered World War II. My parents, who married shortly after graduating from high school, were excited to be starting a family but also justifiably concerned about the impact the war might have on their immediate future. Their anxieties became real concerns when my father felt compelled to enlist in the army in 1943. One of my earliest memories was riding on a train to Anniston, Alabama with my mother for an extended visit with Dad, who was then stationed at Fort McClellan. We stayed in a rented room in a family home in Anniston until Dad received his orders to depart for Europe, and then we traveled back to Illinois to live with my grandmother and grandfather and their teenage daughter, Rose.

By the early 1940s, the US economy was strong because of the demands for supplies and weapons for the war. In fact, so many men were enlisted and serving abroad, there were more opportunities for employment than workers to fill them. As a consequence, women began taking jobs that would have been socially unthinkable just a few years earlier. Like other young women in her situation, Mom decided it would be far better to be working for her country than sitting at home worrying! She quickly found employment welding bomb casings in a factory in Hannibal, Missouri, a small city on the Mississippi River about eighteen miles from where we were living. The work was exacting because imperfections in the welded seams could cause the bombs to detonate prematurely, taking American lives. My mother was mechanically gifted, so she learned her job quickly and evidently did it very well. She was also thrilled to be providing additional income for our needs.

The tenor of those times was very different than that of our present era. The very real threat to our security united Americans with a singleness of purpose, a determination to win, and a cooperative spirit that is difficult to imagine now. While many men and women voluntarily risked their lives to serve abroad, those who remained stateside worked diligently and cooperatively to produce goods and supplies for the war and for the needs at home. At times, necessities such as rubber for tires, gasoline, meat, and sugar were in short supply and had to be rationed. To supplement their food supply, many Americans started raising their own vegetables in small "victory gardens" on their properties or vacant lots. Everyone knew this was a war we simply could not afford to lose.

On the negative side, those left at home also had to deal with nagging uncertainties, powerful fears, and far too often, devastating grief. Because so many young men and women were deployed abroad, a large percentage of the civilian population continually had friends or loved ones at risk of injury, going missing in action, or being killed in battle. Their anxieties and apprehensions were intensified by the exasperating slowness of communication (days, weeks, or even months by mail). In addition, there was always a kind of generalized anxiety about the final outcome of the war. One could never be completely certain that America and its allies would win. Of course, the hardest blows of all were dealt by the dreaded notices that one's worst fears had been realized.

Like many others in her situation, my mother resolved to remain strong, work hard, and save her money. She was eventually able to buy a well-used Model A Ford, which she affectionately nick-named "Old Put Put Bang." It was balky and noisy, but it would reliably get her from point A to point B, and that was all she required of it. Mom had to wear leather clothing on her job, as well as a welder's hood, to protect herself from sparks. I can still remember watching her lace up her leather boots, which came right up to her knees, before she left for work each morning.

For me, life was good in those early years, even though Dad was away and Mom worked. At the time, I was an only child and grandchild, so I received a lot of love and attention. My grandmother was a beauty operator who cut, curled, and coiffed women's hair in her own shop in her home. It was fascinating to watch her work. I vividly remember the very strange-looking apparatus mounted to the ceiling above the beauty chair, which she sometimes used to give permanents (permanent curls or waves). Numerous curlers were attached by wires to this ceiling device. Grandma would apply a lotion to her client's hair, roll up the hair on these curlers, and then flip a switch. Electricity passing through the rollers generated the heat needed to set the curls permanently. By the time Mom and I moved in, this device was outdated, but Grandma was convinced that it was still the best technique for certain styles and types of hair, so she continued to use it.

I looked forward to clients who brought their children with them, because that provided playmates. I also enjoyed spending time with my Aunt Rose. It was really fun when she or Mom would push me in the backyard swing. That swing was hung from a very high limb on a huge old walnut tree. It traversed such a long arc and swung me so high that I could hardly endure the excitement or the relentless tickling in my stomach.

Another fond memory was watching for my Grandpa Dover to come home from work. He was a foreman over a crew that maintained electric lines for the Rural Electric Association in our area. The garage where he stowed the truck at the end of each day was less than a block from the house, so Grandma would often "put me to work" watching for Grandpa. (It also kept me out of the kitchen while she was busy preparing dinner.) Grandpa was always glad to see me and would unfailingly greet me with loving, boisterous excitement.

My father made it through the war without serious physical injury, and after he returned, he rented a small farmhouse for us to live in. One of my early memories there included climbing up by my dad on the couch and listening to him strumming his guitar and singing country and western songs. I also remember when Dad and his younger brothers would skate together on the frozen pond on the property. Another fond memory was playing in the yard with my only consistent playmate (and guardian), an Irish Setter named Tucker.

There were some good memories at that house but also some very upsetting ones. Mom and Dad had both changed significantly during their years apart, and shortly after they were reunited, they started having serious arguments. Dad was drinking heavily, and this created trouble. As the arguments escalated, so did his drinking. He started going out virtually every night and couldn't keep a steady job. Then he started getting physically abusive. My mother was strong and independent and soon decided she had had enough. I still remember the warm summer day when she made the decision to leave. (I was about five at the time.) Mom was visibly upset but resolute. We packed some of our belongings and carried them with us, walking together down the dusty gravel road to a neighbor's house so Mom could use their telephone to call her parents to come and get us in their car.

At that point, we moved back to Grandma and Grandpa's house. My mother was pregnant with my younger sister and wasn't quite sure what to do next. A few weeks after our move, a woman carrying a baby came to Grandma's house and knocked on the front door. She was looking for Dad, claiming that he was the father of her baby and wanting him to pay child support. With this information, Mom filed for divorce and Dad fled to Montana to escape the mess that he had created. I didn't realize it at the time, but from the day he left, I would only see him alive once more in my lifetime, when I was thirty-five with three children of my own. After my sister, Barbara, was born, Mom found a good job at the local post office, and rented "half a house" for us to live in. Grandma lived only a few blocks away, so she continued to help with babysitting and making sure I got to school.

When I was eight and my sister was two, Mom married a local farmer, who was twenty years older than she and who had never married. Orin was a generous and intelligent man, with a droll sense of humor. He loved our mother and had willingly offered to provide the best life he could for all of us. However, Orin was also haunted by feelings of personal inadequacy and betrayal and was locked into a dependent and very frustrating relationship with his parents. As a consequence, he was prone to unpredictable (and sometimes dangerous) outbursts of anger. These episodes and the dark moods that accompanied them became a serious source of strife and trouble in our family.

When Orin met Mom, he was about fifty years behind the times in his farming techniques and his way of life. In large part, this was due to a shortage of cash and his parents' unwillingness to partner with him to invest in more up-to-date equipment. In part, it may also have been due to preference. Orin had a love of history and a deep appreciation for some of the older ways of doing things. Whatever the reason, the farm was never very productive, so he had to borrow money regularly to keep it operating, and then he struggled to repay his debts. Consequently, we learned to live on a very modest income.

For the first three years, we lived in a rented house because the farmhouse that Orin had lived in was old, small, and seriously out of date (no electricity, telephone, running water, or bathroom).

However, renting was costly, so Mom eventually agreed to move to the farm anyway. Orin did some remodeling prior to our move, but it was still a year before we even had electricity. Our heat came from a woodstove, and the wood for fuel came from dead or diseased trees that Orin cut from wooded areas on the farm. We pumped our water by hand from a cistern located just outside the kitchen door and carried it into the house in a bucket. When we wanted a drink of water, we would simply drink from the shared dipper that always hung on the side of the water bucket.

The lack of "modern" conveniences meant we had to do a lot of extra work, and I used to grumble about that. However, as an adult, I was grateful to have learned how people accomplished life in a much earlier time. It was difficult to read, study, or do much else by the dim light of coal-oil lamps, so I learned to finish my homework while there was still daylight. Without electric lights anywhere near, it could get incredibly dark at night. That was particularly scary when I and my younger sister had to make late-night visits to the outhouse. Our little flashlight illuminated only a small area directly ahead of where we were walking, and it was easy to imagine all sorts of dangers lurking in the darkness.

Still, that darkness did have one benefit. I remember staring up in wonder at the night sky and marveling at the uncountable sweep of stars blazing in all their glory. In moments like those, I would sense that there must be a God and that He must be far greater than anything we could imagine. My sister and I loved to go outside on clear summer nights, lay on our backs, and just look up at the stars. We would watch for "shooting stars" and then exclaim excitedly to one another when we spotted one. Sometimes Mom and Orin would join us in our vigils.

By the time we moved to the farm, Orin had purchased a small Ferguson tractor; however, he still did some of the farming on his hilly, red-clay fields with work horses. These were very large, strong animals compared to racing or riding horses, but they were also gentle and well trained. Even with the new tractor, Orin wasn't in any hurry to part with his horses because he had to use them several times to rescue his tractor after it mired down in the wet, sticky clay.

As the oldest child, I was called upon to do many chores. One of these was to milk the cows (before and after school) and another was to help gather (or "shuck") wagonloads of corn from the fields for our pigs and cattle. Orin didn't own a mechanical corn picker, so much of his corn would still be standing in the fields long past fall harvest. When we needed more corn, Orin would hitch up a team of horses that would pull a wagon along the rows of corn. Once in the field, two or three of us (usually Mom, Orin, and I) would walk down the rows, side by side, each assigned two or more rows to shuck.

Removing the corn from the husks and the stalk could be done very efficiently with a little practice. With the aid of a metal "shucking peg," strapped onto our right hands, we would first rip back about half the dried corn husks on an ear with our right hand, pull back the remaining husks with the left hand, pop the ear off the stalk with both hands and fling it into the wagon. The far side of the wagon was fitted with an extension that made it twice as high as the near side That way, ears of corn that flew too high would not just sail over the wagon (and have to be retrieved) but would hit the "bump board" and bounce into the wagon. After we had all shucked from a position slightly behind the wagon up toward the front of it, Orin, would merely command the horses, "Get up," and they would obediently pull the wagon forward another few feet, stop, and wait for the next command. When the fields started thawing in the spring, hand shucking could provide a serious workout. The wet clay would stick to our boots with unbelievable persistence. After every few steps, we would have to stop and vigorously kick the heavy accumulation off our boots before proceeding.

Washing clothes for a family without electricity, a washing machine, a water heater, or indoor plumbing was also a full day's work. We would begin by loading up the heating stove with wood, get a good fire going, place a large metal container called a boiler on top of the stove, and haul in buckets of water from the cistern to be heated. The hot water had to be dipped back out of the boiler (carefully) and transported by bucket to the wash tub. Mom would then scrub each piece of laundry on a scrub board with laundry soap, wring out the soapy water, and rinse the items in a second tub of cool water. After another wringing, we would carry the laundry outside in a large basket and hang it out to dry.

On warm sunny days, this was a pleasant task. However, adverse weather conditions could complicate washday incredibly. On windy days, a clothesline would sometimes break, dumping the clean, wet laundry on the ground, necessitating rewashing and rehanging. Winter was also a challenge. We had to hang clothes quickly and keep warming our hands to avoid frostbite. In addition, the clothes, sheets, and towels would freeze on the line, forming stiff shapes that waved in the breeze like giant pieces of cardboard before they finally dried and softened. When we were finally able to afford electricity and a washing machine, washday became much easier.

After we moved to the farm, life settled down to a predictable routine. There was always a lot of work because we depended upon the farm for all our income and much of our food. In the spring, we would go out in the woods and pastures to search for morel mushrooms. During the summer, we had peach, apricot, plum, pear, cherry, and apple trees that usually bore an abundance of fruit. We would also go out in the pasture to patches of wild black-berries and gooseberries and pick these in season. And we grew potatoes and many other kinds of vegetables in a very large garden. All of this fruit and produce needed to be cleaned and preserved as the season progressed, so Mom and I spent many hours in the kitchen together preserving food for winter.

Orin had good pasture land on the farm and raised cattle and pigs as well as corn, oats, hay, etc. In addition, Mom always raised chickens. From these we had our own milk, butter, cream, cottage cheese, eggs, and meat. My days were full, but after I got used to the work, I didn't mind. I loved working outside and liked the discipline and feeling of accomplishment that came with the work.

When fall arrived and it was time to go back to school, I had mixed feelings. I truly enjoyed studying and learning new things. Academic work had always been fairly easy, and when I started applying the discipline I was learning at home to my school work, I began earning very high marks. These achievements became a very significant source of encouragement and reinforcement.

It was the prospect of increased social interaction at school that produced mixed feelings. I did have some good friends, and I looked forward to being with them again. However, I never quite fit in with the popular group in my class. I had had a moderate problem with my weight, even since first grade, had been teased, and was very sensitive about that issue. Because money was scarce, my clothes were usually not up to popular standards either. However, I did discover that by working hard and getting top grades, I could still earn a great deal of respect from these peers. Achievement not only gave me a degree of acceptance, but it also boosted my self-esteem. It became a very powerful motivator.

I had had some exposure to Christianity early in my life; however, as a teenager, I did not have enough understanding or commitment to God's greater purposes to help me adopt wiser priorities. While we were living with Grandma, we regularly attended a small local church and I began to learn about God and Jesus and some of the basic tenets of the Christian faith. When Mom moved to her own place, our church attendance became more sporadic, and after she married Orin, who was not a believer, she eventually stopped attending altogether. While my sister and I were young, Mom made sure we recited our bedtime prayers each night and said grace before meals. And at least until I was about thirteen, Mom and Grandma worked together to make sure we could attend Sunday school and church or youth activities at least occasionally.

When I was twelve, my grandmother explained to me that I needed to be saved and to be baptized if I wanted to go to Heaven. I thought about that quite seriously and decided that I did believe that Jesus was God's Son and that I wanted to turn over my life to Him and be baptized. Even though my understanding of salvation at that time was rudimentary, I believe my decision to give my life to Jesus was sincere. I remember receiving a beautiful, new white dress for that occasion and insisting, over Mom's objections, that I wear it right into the water during the baptism. Keeping it back to wear after I was baptized just didn't seem right. That precious dress needed to be committed to Jesus too.

It would have been wonderful if I had been able to hold on to that commitment, but without consistent church attendance, with little grounding in the Bible and an increasing preoccupation with my own plans and goals, my allegiance to Jesus faded. By the time I entered high school, I was very focused upon myself, getting top grades, and impressing other people. I asked for and received permission to take course overloads every year to make sure I was well prepared for college and a possible career in science. I also engaged in a number of extra-curricular activities.

I was able to do very well in my freshman and sophomore years, but this success also went to my head and I became proud and over-confident. During that same time period, Mom and Orin had two children of their own, a boy and a girl. They struggled with this new set of challenges, along with ongoing financial difficulties, and started having long and bitter arguments. My sister and I tried to stay out of these conflicts, but more often than not, one or the other of us would become an irritant because of something we said or did. After a while, I would come home from school hoping that no one would be home. I didn't mind if that meant I was left with extra housework or chores to do because at least I could do those things in peace.

The success and encouragement I was obtaining at school and the painful chaos at home both strongly reinforced my desire to get away, go to college, and "make something of myself." I began to dream of the day when I could leave home, get an education, and begin a prestigious career. Whenever life at home became overwhelming, I would return to these dreams for encouragement. Once in a while, reality would break through, causing me to question how all this was actually going to happen since neither my parents nor anyone else I knew could help me financially. No matter. With youthful overconfidence, I simply assumed that I could earn scholarships or perhaps enlist in some branch of the Armed Services and find an entrance into higher education that way. I just knew that this was something *I* had to do and that somehow *I* would find a way.

These ambitions were at the forefront of my thinking in 1957 when I was sixteen and just beginning my junior year in high school. The school year started well, but in the second week, I became very ill. I was running a high fever and had a lot of muscle pain and a very bad headache. At first, our family doctor thought I had a bad case of influenza. A couple days later, I noticed that at times muscles in my legs would twitch uncontrollably and that both legs were weak. After my second visit to this doctor, when I started down the steps from his office, both of my knees buckled and I fell. Fortunately, Mom was right beside me and was able to catch me and break my fall so I wasn't injured. She helped me up, but I could barely walk.

When the doctor learned how I had fallen, he changed his advice on the spot, deciding that I should go directly to the nearest hospital, in Hannibal, Missouri, for additional tests. When I got to that hospital, I could hardly move my legs and the pain was incredible. A doctor there took some fluid from my spinal cord and soon diagnosed the problem—paralytic poliomyelitis!

That news hit me with explosive force! Suddenly everything that had seemed so important—achievement, physical capability, and plans for my future—shattered into a cloud of tiny pieces and slowly settled into a nondescript pile of debris. Then the news got even scarier. The doctor in Hannibal urged my parents to let him send me, quickly by ambulance, to St. Anthony's Hospital in St. Louis, Missouri, which had special facilities for treating polio cases. I was still running a very high fever, and it wasn't clear how much further the infection would go. If it adversely affected my breathing, I might need a respirator or even an iron lung in order to survive! Mom consented, and she and I were quickly loaded into an ambulance. I was very ill and very sleepy. The only other thing I remember about that trip was alternately sleeping and being awakened by the blaring siren whenever the ambulance passed through towns along the 120-mile journey from Hannibal to St. Louis.

Chapter 4

Unmerited Favor

I t was late afternoon when the ambulance that was transporting me arrived at St. Anthony's Hospital. I was admitted and quickly taken to a room by myself. Nurses stopped by frequently, checking my temperature, my pain levels, and especially my breathing. That evening another young woman, probably in her early twenties, joined me in my room. She too had just been admitted with a diagnosis of polio. I noticed that she could move her legs easily and turn from side to side in bed—feats I could no longer accomplish. That made me very apprehensive because it appeared that I was far worse off than she.

Fortunately, drowsiness overwhelmed my worries and I fell back asleep. I was awakened some time later when attendants came in and moved my roommate out of the room. After an hour or so, they also moved me to a new room. My roommate was there too, but she was now lying in an iron lung and only her head and neck were visible. In addition, a nurse was stationed right beside her.

Periodically I would hear strange gurgling sounds coming from the other side of the room, so I used my arms to shift my position in bed so I could see what was causing the noises. To my horror, I discovered that they were coming from a suctioning apparatus that the nurse used to clear fluids that were accumulating in this woman's throat. The possible implications nearly sent me into a panic—since we both had polio, what was happening to her could also happen to me! As I continued to stare at the apparatus, I noticed something even more alarming. The suction tube was not inserted through her mouth but through a surgical opening in her throat!

The iron lung made regular whooshing sounds as it assisted my roommate's breathing. Between the whooshing, the gurgling, my high fever, and my own very limited ability to move, I became very frightened indeed. Fortunately, I continued to pass the periodic breathing tests throughout the night and never did require oxygen or mechanical assistance to breathe.

Sometime during that night, after I had fallen asleep, my roommate was moved again. When I awoke the next morning, I immediately sensed that something had changed. The room was now very quiet, and neither my roommate nor the iron lung were anywhere in sight. I grew increasingly uneasy but tried to reassure myself that she had probably just been relocated for some reason. After what seemed a very long time, a nurse came in to check on me and I asked her how my former roommate was faring. At first, the nurse was reluctant to answer, but finally she told me that this young woman had died during the night in the iron lung! Unfortunately, she had contracted bulbar polio, which was often fatal. It had taken her life by paralyzing the muscles that enabled her to breathe.

My fever broke sometime the next day. I felt better, but I was still incredibly weak. It was difficult to move my legs, I couldn't turn from side to side, nor could I remain on either side unless supported with pillows. When I was elevated to a sitting position in the hospital bed, I could maintain that position and move my left hand and arm normally, but I had definite weaknesses in my right hand and arm. I could raise the right arm enough to allow me to eat, but not high enough to comb my hair. My right thumb had been weakened, and as if to add insult to injury, when I looked in a mirror, I discovered that my right eyelid was also drooping. Many muscles had been adversely affected, and I didn't know how much I would recover. I was also separated by 120 miles from family and friends. At that time, it appeared that I was going to have to cope with this distressing situation pretty much on my own.

A peculiar incident that occurred the next day served to underscore the potential seriousness of my situation. A television reporter on one of our local stations at home actually announced that I had died during the night! Ironically, an aunt of mine heard this announcement, remained frozen in stunned silence for several seconds, then declared loudly to no one in particular, "I am just not going to believe it!" Mom had called her the night before to tell her I was doing better. So Aunty quickly called Mom, and Mom hurriedly called the hospital just to make sure that I was still among the living.

Our relatives and close friends were all informed of the mistake within a couple of hours, but no one thought to call the principal or teachers at my small local high school. They were actually in the process of collecting money for flowers for my funeral and comforting my classmates when they discovered that I was still very much alive! Fortunately, I didn't learn of this incident until much later, and by that time, I could even see some humor in it. To quote an apt rejoinder made by Samuel Clemens (Mark Twain) after he read an announcement of his own death in a local newspaper, "Reports of my death have been greatly exaggerated!" We never discovered where this error originated, but it's likely that someone at the hospital mistakenly attached my name to my former roommate's outcome, because she did indeed pass away that night.

As I began to recover, it became very obvious that my physical losses were serious. I longed for reassurance and encouragement, so I started asking doctors and nurses if I would get better and whether they thought I would be able to walk again. They all gave me the same answer—they simply didn't know at this early stage of my recovery. With growing alarm, I questioned more persistently. Finally one doctor told me that I would probably get stronger and recover some function, but he didn't think I would ever be able to walk on my own again. That pronouncement was devastating.

In fact, that opinion helped catapult me into a very difficult internal struggle that reached a climax a couple of days later. By that time, I was able to think more clearly and could see for myself that I might not be able to walk again. If I could not walk, obtaining a college education did not seem very plausible either. Without being able to walk, I probably would not be able to work and earn money for college, nor would I be able to enlist in the Armed Services and get an education that way. Then even more disturbing questions began to surface. Would I even be able to live independently and support myself, or would I remain an invalid, forced to live at home, caught in all the discord, even becoming an additional and substantial reason for it? I hated the thought of becoming a financial or physical burden on anyone, especially on my parents.

These possibilities were extremely upsetting, and I couldn't just will them to go away. Afternoon morphed into night. I struggled to get to sleep and then slept fitfully. Sometime after midnight, I awoke feeling very anxious, alone, and helpless. I looked about aimlessly in the dim light, hoping to find something to distract my thoughts and to relieve my anxieties. My gaze eventually came to rest on a crucifix hanging on the wall opposite my bed. That stirred memories of church and my earlier commitment to Jesus. I had felt confident of my faith then, but that night in the hospital, I wasn't sure what I believed.

After being baptized, I had attended church infrequently. Pretty much on my own and without a biblical understanding of the Christian life or a strong commitment to living it, I had strayed badly. In fact, by the time polio struck, I had begun to question my faith and the truth of the Bible. I was full of pride, overconfident, hooked on achieving success, and determined to live my own way. However, putting my way first rather than God's way had created one big mess.

My overconfidence had lured me into putting off getting the simple vaccination that would have prevented polio altogether. My inflated ego and critical spirit had fueled harsh and damaging conflicts with both parents. Still worse, my poor judgment and lack of self-discipline had led me headlong into an impulsive romantic liaison with our hired man, who was addicted to alcohol and deeply troubled psychologically. Continuing in that relationship would have been disastrous. As I would recognize later, God, through polio, "worked for my good" in two ways here (see Romans 8:28). He opened my eyes to the folly and sinfulness of that relationship and forcefully removed me from it.

Unpleasant memories, thoughts, regrets, and fears kept playing and replaying in my mind, making me even more depressed. My attention shifted back to the crucifix, and I began to think about Jesus. As I did, I sensed a faint stirring of hope. "Maybe Jesus is real." "Maybe He actually does love me." "Maybe He will forgive me and help me find purpose in my life again." I vacillated back and forth for a while, but deep inside, I knew what I needed to do. Finally I simply prayed, "Jesus, I am very sorry I have drifted away and doubted You. Now I am in deep trouble and I cannot help myself. If You are real, I give You my life for whatever it may now be worth." My prayer was marred by doubts and pride, and I don't know if my repentance was actually genuine, but it was all I knew to do at the time and the Lord graciously accepted it. That night, I felt a sense of peace and was assured that I was not alone. I did not know what my life would be like, but I was able to leave my future in God's hands that night and rest.

A few days after that prayer, I began to see definite signs that something unusual was happening and dared to hope that it might be from God. One powerful indication occurred on my first day of physical therapy. My new therapist, Mrs. Miller, was a beautiful, gentle young woman with deep-blue eyes, jet-black hair, and a caring, serene disposition. I liked her immediately. That day I had therapy in a "Hubbard Tank," a human-sized, oddly shaped container that was filled with warm circulating water. I was transferred from a cart onto a stretcher, and the stretcher was lowered into the tank. Mrs. Miller explained that I would start therapy by doing exercises in water because the water would allow my weakened muscles to move more easily. Some muscles that were too weak to move against the force of gravity while I was lying on a mat could produce quite a bit of movement if assisted by the buoyancy of the water. She was right. In the water, I was able to move my legs in ways that I could not manage in bed.

I should have been elated to discover that there was some capability for movement left in those leg muscles, but instead I just felt very depressed because the muscles were so weak. We tried some different exercises, but Mrs. Miller could see that I was getting emotional and was just not motivated to keep on trying. She chided me gently, telling me that if I wanted to regain strength, I was going to have to work for it. And then she made the comment that she *understood* how I felt. Right then, in a sudden flash of anger that surprised both of us, I asked her how she could possibly understand how it felt to be so incapacitated—she was so obviously strong and physically fit. She responded firmly but gently, "But I do know what this is like. I too had paralytic polio that affected my legs and trunk muscles. I too was told that I would probably never walk. But I did not give up. My mother and I worked together on my exercise program for years, and now I am as strong as you see today!"

Her response completely surprised and disarmed me. I simply didn't know I had any chance of regaining so much strength. I had concluded that I couldn't recover very much, so it took me a few moments to begin to grasp the incredible implications of what she had said. The possibility of such recovery, in the light of what I had assumed was permanent loss, was completely overwhelming, and I burst into tears! After I regained my composure, I apologized to Mrs. Miller, thanked her sincerely for her encouragement, and determined in my heart to start working as hard for physical recovery as I had for grades.

It wasn't until a little later, after the therapy session, that I began to grasp just how significant our new relationship actually was. How was it possible, I wondered, that I should have a therapist so like me, fairly close to me in age, who had sustained very similar neurological damage from paralytic polio, but who had also completely overcome it? How many physical therapists in St. Louis, or even in the entire United States, had even had paralytic polio or, if they had, were able to prevail over its effects so completely that they could become physical therapists? Surely this convergence between Mrs. Miller's life and my own couldn't be just a coincidence; the probabilities seemed far too small. But if this wasn't coincidence, the only other explanation I could think of was that it must be from God, perhaps in answer to my prayer. He knew that I would need strong encouragement to recover and was showing me, through Mrs. Miller, that there was still much hope for my future.

Before long, other encouraging signs began to appear as well. With time and regular exercise, quite a few of the muscles in my legs, back, and abdomen started regaining strength. I was soon able to transfer in and out of a manual wheelchair by myself and, with it, to travel to any area of the hospital on my own. After about three weeks of therapy, Mrs. Miller had me try to get up and stand just holding on to two parallel bars. These were two sturdy metal handrails, each about ten feet long, that were parallel to each other, about thirty inches apart, and attached to the floor. They were designed to enable patients with weak legs and strong arms to walk by supporting some of their weight with their arms.

On my first attempt, I was able to stand, unassisted, holding on to the bars. Then Mrs. Miller asked me to try to take some steps. By using the handrails and shifting a lot of my weight to my arms, I was able to walk down to the end of the bars and back, although I had to push my knees back into an unnatural "locking" position to keep them from buckling under the remaining weight of my body. This accomplishment elated both of us because it was an early and strong indication that one day I would probably be able to walk fairly normally again!

In addition to these encouraging developments, there were powerful indications that the Lord was providing for my other needs. One big problem I faced while recovering was my inability to attend school. I had just begun my junior year in high school when polio struck, and it was soon obvious that I wouldn't be able to go back to school anytime soon. Fortunately, Mom and my teachers devised a workable solution for this problem. My teachers sent my assignments via mail or with Mom, and after I completed them, I returned them for grading. My tests and quizzes were proctored by the kindly nun who supervised our floor. I was also able to continue my typing class by practicing on an electric typewriter in the occupational therapy room (which also provided needed exercise for my right hand and thumb). Because I was given all of this generous assistance, I was able to catch up and then keep up with my classes during my entire three-and-a-half month stay in the hospital!

A second issue, which could have created an impossible burden for my parents, was the cost of my medical treatment. The specialized treatment I received plus the sheer length of my stay at the hospital racked up an enormous bill. Fortunately, and I can only say by the Lord's provision, Mom was told when I was admitted that because my diagnosis was poliomyelitis, all of my medical bills would be paid by the March of Dimes Foundation! This organization was founded in 1938 by President Franklin Delano Roosevelt to help victims and their families cope with the regular polio epidemics that swept across our country at that time. (Roosevelt himself had been a victim of paralytic polio before becoming president.) The foundation's purpose was to fund polio research and to help pay for the extended treatment and equipment required by polio patients. Most of the money that financed this huge project was generously donated by American citizens.

When I contracted polio in 1957, the Salk polio vaccine had been available for about three years. The first inoculations were given only to young children who were at the greatest risk. Later, when there was enough vaccine for everyone and it was offered for free right at my high school, I was busy and foolishly skipped that opportunity, thinking I would get it the next time around. However, before I had that next opportunity, I was struck by the disease myself. At that time, the number of new polio cases across the country had already dropped precipitously. In 1953, there about 35,000 cases of polio in the United States. When I was admitted in 1957, the number of cases nationwide had dropped to 5,600, and by 1961, there were only 161 reported cases in the entire country.

To help me appreciate the amazing effectiveness of the new vaccine, the nun who supervised our floor once took me up to see the hospital's cavernous attic, where they stored unused equipment. I will never forget entering that space in my wheelchair and seeing endless row after endless row of iron lungs, which by that time were no longer needed. That was a very sobering and thought-provoking experience. Those machines, along with the memory of my former roommate's fatal struggle with polio in one of them, made me very grateful to be alive, to be breathing normally, and to have the physical capability I had retained.

With continued physical therapy, I kept regaining strength, although the quadriceps muscles in both legs and some muscles in my lower back and abdomen remained fairly weak. The way I had to lock my knees to walk prompted the orthopedic doctor to order long leg braces and crutches for me to use. He anticipated that walking this way without the braces would eventually damage my knees. The braces were also meant to keep my knees from buckling unexpectedly, causing me to fall. However, walking with them meant I had to swing one leg forward, move a crutch, swing the other leg forward, move the other crutch, etc. Walking this way was slow and cumbersome, and the braces also made it very difficult to get in and out of my wheelchair. I really disliked using them. Fortunately, I didn't have to do it very long.

By mid-November, Mrs. Miller and my doctors decided that I was strong enough to make a three-day home visit over Thanksgiving.

I was grateful for the opportunity but also apprehensive about how I would manage at home. The hospital loaned me a wheelchair, but I knew it wouldn't be very useful because our house was small and crowded. We also had steps at both entrances, so I knew I would need considerable help just to get in and out of the house. In addition, we didn't have indoor plumbing. All we had was the old outhouse several yards from the house. When I did get home, the physical challenges were substantial, but Mom was strong and very resourceful, and working together, we were able to figure out how to manage my basic needs. She was a very significant source of support and encouragement on that visit.

It was my stepfather's reactions that were hard to deal with. Orin had only visited me once, early on, at the hospital in St. Louis, and since that time had been hearing how much I was improving. So he was not prepared for the degree of disability that he observed when he had to help me get into the house in the wheelchair or when he watched my awkward attempts to use the chair, crutches, and braces in very inaccessible spaces. After all that I had been able to do physically before polio, I undoubtedly looked pretty helpless. Every once in a while in unguarded moments, I noticed that he was looking at me with sadness and pity, shaking his head as if in disbelief or uncertainty about what to say or do.

Orin was unusually quiet for the first two days of my visit and finally spoke to me seriously a couple of hours before Mom and I had to leave for St. Louis. I am sure he meant to encourage me, and in retrospect, he was being generous. However, when he finally spoke, the implications of his words undercut my hopes for recovery and a meaningful life like a knife. "Betty, I know you aren't going to be able to do much around here anymore. You can't help with the outside work or chores like you used to, but I will let you stay here anyway. Maybe you can help out a little with housework or taking care of your little brother and sister." Unfortunately, what I heard in my heart was, "Polio has wrecked your life and you are not going to get better. You are pretty worthless now because you can't work, but I will give you a place to live. Perhaps you can repay me by doing what little you can." I think I managed to stammer a half-hearted "Thank you" instead of getting totally depressed or defensive, but I was really glad that it was about time to leave.

Fortunately, even in the face that discouraging conversation and other challenges, the Lord continued to reveal His love and faithfulness to me by granting me a great deal of physical recovery. My recovery wasn't sudden or complete, as in a supernatural, New Testament healing. However, in retrospect, and with a much greater appreciation for the incredible *natural* powers of healing that God has built into our bodies, that recovery seems nothing short of a miracle to me now.

In my case, unlike its effects on Ken, polio did not completely destroy the motor neurons to any affected muscle group in my body. With time and exercise, the motor neurons that survived branched extensively to re-enervate nearby muscle fibers that had lost their connection with the nervous system. As a result, I eventually regained almost all of my strength in many of the muscles that had been weakened and at least some movement and strength in the rest.

I was permanently discharged from St. Anthony's Hospital shortly before Christmas of 1957. Mom learned how to help me with the physical therapy I needed and readily agreed to bring me back for occasional outpatient follow-ups. When I left the hospital, I took my braces and my crutches but not a wheelchair because my walking was improving and the wheelchair wouldn't be very useful anyway. Once at home, I discovered that I did not need the crutches or braces because I no longer needed to lock my knees to walk. I was able to walk from place to place in the house, occasionally just using furniture or counters for a little extra support. Eventually I was able to walk independently indoors and use one short crutch, which functioned somewhat like a cane, when I walked for longer distances, navigated uneven terrain, or had to climb up steps or curbs.

By February of my junior year, I was able to return to high school because the principal moved all of my classes to the first floor and Mom and Orin provided my transportation. By September of my senior year, I was able to manage the steps into the school bus and to climb the stairs at school using my crutch. The one problem that persisted, for as long as I was able to walk, was the ease with which I could fall. If I stumbled slightly or tripped, I would fall hard, usually landing on my knees. I didn't have much strength in the muscles that could have helped me regain my balance or break my fall. Those falls were painful, but later, after I had fully surrendered my life to Jesus, they also served to remind me that I was not self-sufficient—my strength and ability to continue to function was a gift from the Lord.

During my last year and a half at home, I continued to work hard on my studies, continued to get good grades, and still had a very strong desire to go to college. However, realistically, in light of our financial situation and my physical disabilities, I just couldn't see how this was going to happen. Yet the Lord also opened this door for me in some totally unexpected ways.

Early in my senior year (1958-59), my high-school physics teacher approached two of us in class to ask if we would like to compete with other high-school seniors across the country in a new science competition called the Westinghouse Science Talent Search. This was just one of several vigorous public and private initiatives taking place at that time to find and train more American scientists and engineers. These initiatives were a response to Russia's launch of Sputnik, the first satellite to orbit the earth, on October 10, 1957. At that time, our country was locked in the Cold War arms race with Russia, so Russia's impressive achievement was interpreted as a serious and immediate threat because it suggested that Russia was way ahead of us in space technology. The thinking at that time was that our country needed to catch up fast, and the best way to do that was to train more scientists.

For the Westinghouse competition, students were required to take tests that measured their general aptitude and knowledge of science and to design an original science experiment, run it, and report the results. I took on this challenge, not really appreciating the odds against me or the disadvantage of attending a small, rural high school, which had only very basic scientific equipment to work with. Yet as it turned out, this limitation didn't really matter. The experiment I believe the Lord brought to my mind didn't need high-tech equipment. It was based on a simple paper-and-pencil puzzle in which there were three houses (represented as three squares in a row) and three utilities (represented by three circles in a row below the squares). The challenge was to draw lines that would connect each house to each utility without crossing any lines or rights-of-way.

This cannot be done. I accepted that conclusion but was curious about why it could not be done and what might happen if one varied the number of houses or utilities or represented the problem in three dimensions as opposed to drawing on a sheet of paper. I did a series of experiments varying these conditions systematically, drew pictures of the solutions for each (when there was a solution), and discovered a simple equation that predicted some of the outcomes. For the three-dimensional experiments, I constructed models with cubes and spheres of modeling clay to represent houses and utilities, connecting these with short pieces of dynamite wire (which came with different colored plastic coatings, was thin and flexible, and was readily available). Not surprisingly, I took some good-natured teasing from my science teacher about my low-tech equipment. Somewhat grandly and with little understanding of what I might be implying, I entitled my report "An Experiment in Abstract Mathematics" and sent it off.

Amazingly to me (and to my science teacher), I was selected as a winner along with thirty-nine other students across Illinois. I found out later that my "experiment" was actually an experimental approach to a sophisticated problem in a branch of mathematics called topology! As I look back at this turn of events now, I can see that much of my opportunity for a college education was initiated with a brain teaser, some clay, dynamite wire, and some carefully placed guidance from the Lord. Surely our God can make much out of little!

The names of the award winners were publicized widely among various colleges and universities, and I soon started receiving letters from many schools inviting me to apply. Shortly after that, I received notice that I had qualified for a state scholarship that would potentially pay for all four years of tuition at any college in Illinois. Then I received a letter from our local state representative, telling me about the State Rehabilitation Program in Illinois and letting me know that this program would probably pay for the rest of my college expenses. This letter was remarkable because the representative did not know me and did not realize that I was disabled until he learned this from a separate article in our local newspaper.

I applied for and received the additional support I still needed from the State Rehabilitation Program. Then, with all the financial resources in place and still a bit disoriented by this rapid and amazing turn of events, I received notice from the admissions department at the University of Illinois at Champaign-Urbana that I had been accepted and had also been named a "James Scholar" in a new, university-wide honors program that had just been put into place!

This was all very heady stuff; it came very fast, and I scarcely knew what to make of it. Looking back, it is very clear to me that the Lord was orchestrating these events. Even at the time, this thought did occur to me. However, I had not yet fully committed my life to the Lord and did not give God the credit or thanks He deserved. Instead I surmised that I must be getting all this opportunity and recognition because I had unusual ability! It was with this mindset, once again overconfident and filled with pride, that I began making preparations for my freshman year at the University of Illinois.

Chapter 5

Converging Pathways

I arrived at the University of Illinois in late August of 1959 with great expectations. There were new people to meet, interesting places to see, and exciting things to do. I was very grateful for the opportunity to be there and confident that a college education would help me find the better life I was longing for.

Because of my physical disability, I was automatically placed in the Rehabilitation Program. This remarkable program was established in 1948 by Dr. Timothy Nugent after he learned of the frustration of disabled veterans returning from World War II who couldn't take advantage of their education benefits in the GI Bill of Rights simply because the sidewalks and buildings on college campuses were not accessible for wheelchairs. He quickly realized that this was also a problem for civilians with disabilities, and that it was something that could and should be changed.

Tim Nugent was very energetic and resourceful, and he advocated tirelessly for programs like this until his retirement in 1985. With great persistence, he persuaded reluctant officials and trustees at the U of I to invest in curb cuts, ramps, elevators, and larger bathrooms so the sidewalks and all the classrooms were accessible. He also made sure there were accessible dormitory rooms and obtained funding for two large buses that were furnished with wheelchair lifts and tie-downs so students in the program could get from class to class on the sprawling campus. The program also had its own building, offering physical therapy and exercise equipment that students used to meet their physical education requirements. I was delighted to learn that I could meet my requirements with individually supervised swimming lessons.

That fall, before classes started, all of the students in the program were invited to a picnic at a lake in a nearby state park. We all loaded into the special buses and enjoyed the food, games, boat rides, and a time to get acquainted. On the way back, someone on our bus started singing old camp songs and the rest of us joined in. It was an encouraging beginning for the semester ahead.

Before I could sign up for classes that semester, I had to meet with an adviser. Since I had indicated an interest in majoring in physics and had been placed in the new James Scholars program, I was assigned to a professor in that department rather than a regular counselor. He had not advised freshmen before and had apparently assumed that I was incredibly capable because he recommended that I take twenty hours my first semester (compared to the recommended load of sixteen hours), with sixteen of those hours in honors classes. Overconfidence trumped my initial reservations, and I went along with his suggestions. That was not a good decision.

In high school, I had been able to take course overloads, engage in extracurricular activities, meet responsibilities at home, and still maintain high grades. However, the honors-level classes at the U of I were much more demanding than any I had taken. In addition, I still had much to learn about interacting with peers. I hadn't had much opportunity for this in high school, aside from the time I spent in school, in extracurricular activities, or on the school bus. On campus, it was easy to make new friends and to go and do things together. I was also surprised and pleased when I started getting requests for dates (which had happened only once in high school). So for a while, it was difficult to refuse any of these requests even though they did cut into time I needed for study.

My new life with its abundant social interactions was incredibly satisfying, and it was often difficult for me to attend to my work. I tried, but with these other interests, I simply could not keep up with the demands of all five classes. I began falling behind and not doing well on assignments. About a third of the way through the semester, I finally withdrew from one four-hour course and that helped, but by then it was still a struggle to try to catch up in the other four. By the end of the semester I had managed a D in my math class and B's and C's in the rest—not a good start for an honors student. I went home for Christmas break feeling down and thoroughly deflated.

When I returned for the second semester, I had a normal course load and a more realistic estimate of the time and effort needed for study. I was still troubled by the discrepancy between my apparent successes in high school and my poor first-semester grades at the university. Three reasons for the disparity were obvious: an overambitious schedule, inadequate study skills, and the choice to use a lot of time for socializing. However, deep down, I also started questioning whether I was really as capable as I had so fondly imagined. Later, after fully accepting Jesus as Lord and Savior, I realized that I had actually had little influence over the final events that allowed me to attend the U of I. In actuality, it was God who made those things happen. He simply had a purpose for my life that required an education and provided an extraordinary way for me to attain it.

As I became acquainted with advisors and teachers, I also began to question my assumption that an education and a successful career were foolproof paths to happiness and meaning. The educated people around me didn't seem any happier than people I knew who didn't have a college education. In fact, some of them seemed more dissatisfied and pessimistic. This was particularly evident in classes where professors pushed Darwinian evolution as an explanation for human origins. If they were right and we all came into being by accident, our lives were indeed hopeless and meaningless. Having a prestigious career did not seem to translate into a living a better life, either. I observed a lot of envy, pride, and posturing among my professors, and it didn't take long to learn of professors who had abandoned their wives to consort with younger and more attractive college women.

As I thought about those things and struggled with my own beliefs, I became mildly depressed. If life actually had no meaning and we had no real purpose for all of our striving and hard work, why bother? Eventually, on the advice of a friend, I contacted the student counseling center and went in for a few counseling sessions to see if these would help, but they didn't. Fortunately, sheer busyness came to my aid. As the demands of the semester grew, I had less time to think about these troubling issues and simply settled down to work. I received better grades the second semester, and that was an encouragement.

By the time I arrived on campus for my sophomore year, in September of 1960, I definitely had a more realistic perspective. A good education and a rewarding career were not guarantees of happiness or fulfillment; however, working hard and trying to accomplish personal goals were still intrinsically rewarding, and I did need to earn a living, so continuing on and working diligently seemed the best thing to do. I decided to trim back social activities and dating and put my studies first. My new roommate, Jan, was a good friend, and we shared the same academic goals.

Unbeknownst to me, while Jan and I were getting settled in our dorm room, Ken was driving from Chicago to the University of Illinois to begin his doctoral studies. He still felt somewhat conflicted about whether or not he was doing the right thing. After he arrived and discovered that he had been placed in the Rehabilitation Program without his prior knowledge and was required to include regular physical therapy sessions in his schedule and live in an undergraduate dormitory, he was really irritated.

Ken, who was thirty at the time, had been counting on having his own room, off campus, where he would always have a quiet place to study and to work for the university in his new position as a graduate assistant. It appeared to him that he was being treated like an undergraduate simply because he was disabled. Ken was so frustrated that he was about ready to cancel his plans, turn around, and drive right back to Chicago. Still, something inside told him to calm down and not to act in haste, so he hit the pause button and examined his circumstances more thoroughly.

As he did so, Ken learned that there were actually many advantages with this arrangement. For one, the dormitory he would be living in had its own spacious cafeteria, and his room and the bathrooms on his floor were fully wheelchair accessible. Ken could park his car right outside the entrance to that dormitory, and since virtually all the sidewalks and buildings were accessible, he could also use his wheelchair to get around campus rather than driving, trying to find a place to park, and then walking to his destination with his crutches and braces. It also encouraged him to learn that he would be rooming with another older graduate student who was also in the Rehab Program. Ken's dorm was close to the Rehab Center and the departure area for the special buses, so he could easily use his wheelchair and take advantage of that service to get around on campus. Although he was not aware of it at the time, there was another important reason for him to remain at the U of I, stay in the dorm, and use the buses. We eventually met each other on a Rehab bus!

The morning we met, just a week or so into the fall semester, Ken was already on the bus in his wheelchair when I boarded via the steps using my crutch. I saw him looking at me rather intently, so I smiled, said, "Hi, how are you doing" (or something like that), and walked back to a seat and sat down, mostly thinking about my next class. Ken was very curious about me and was surprised to see me get on the bus using a crutch. He had seen me a few days earlier with my roommate, Jan, pushing her in her wheelchair. At the time, he wondered who I was and why I was pushing the chair for her, not realizing that I too was disabled. What Ken didn't know was that Jan allowed me to push her wheelchair when we were going to the Rehab Center together. That way I didn't have to take my crutch because her wheelchair handles gave me extra support when I needed it. I was able to push the wheelchair easily on level, paved surfaces, but when pushing became more difficult (e.g., going up a hill), Jan would quickly assist.

Ken told me much later (after we were married and I had fully accepted the Lord myself) that he was deeply attracted to me when he saw me on the bus and that was why he kept staring. Moreover, while he was staring, he had the clear sense that the Lord was speaking to him, letting him know that I was the person he was going to marry! This really astonished Ken for two reasons. For one, he hadn't even been thinking about the possibility of dating or getting married. Second, the only other time that he had received such a clear message from the Lord was in his crisis with polio at the hospital, when he was assured that he would live and would have a very meaningful life. This second experience really shook him up. He had come to the U of I with one goal in mind, to earn a PhD and then return to Argonne. This new information forced him to rethink many of his prior assumptions about his future.

At first, Ken simply kept this experience to himself and started praying about it. Later he shared it with his mother, Elsie, and asked her to pray about it too. Over the next several weeks, we occasionally met on the bus and engaged in polite conversation. In the meantime, Ken was seeking assurance that this experience was truly from the Lord and evaluating whether he could be an adequate husband, provider, and possibly, parent.

After he was sure that this was indeed from the Lord, he called and asked me if I would go out with him for dinner and to see a movie. As a nineteen-year-old sophomore, I was quite flattered to be asked for a date by a doctoral student, and I was so used to interacting with other disabled students that I wasn't particularly concerned that I had only seen Ken in a wheelchair. However, that evening, I saw him in a completely different light. Ken picked me up at my dorm in his car, a sharp-looking 1957 Plymouth Belvedere that he had purchased shortly before he began working at Argonne. It sported prominent tail fins and plenty of chrome, and I was duly impressed. I was also impressed by the way Ken managed getting seated, getting up, and walking with his crutches and braces. In spite of his obvious physical disability, he was independent, self-confident, and very much in control of the situation. I could tell right away this was one very strong and determined man.

In the restaurant that night, we discovered that we had a number of things in common in addition to the fact that our physical disabilities were due to polio. Our areas of training and interest overlapped a great deal, and since Ken was still fascinated with agriculture, he was delighted to learn that I had been raised on a farm. He plied me with questions about our crops, animals, acreage, crop yields, and so on.

The movie Ken had chosen for us to see that evening was "Ben Hur," which had distinct Christian themes running through it. In retrospect, I think one reason he chose this particular movie was so he could gauge my reaction to it and find out in discussion afterward whether or not I was a Christian. I did not know Ken's beliefs at the time, and when the issue arose, I told him quite honestly that I wasn't sure what I believed. I had had experiences that made me think that there was a God and that Jesus was real, but I also had significant doubts. At that time I was leaning toward agnosticism, and what I was hearing from professors and some other students simply reinforced that perspective. Ken was a strong Christian, so I am sure my words created a lot of dissonance. However, he never made this a big issue, nor did he stop dating me.

Our second date was less formal. We stopped for a hamburger at a "Steak and Shake" and went to a drive-in theater. Ken could have saved some money by just finding a place where we could park and talk because we were soon so involved in conversation that Ken turned off the speaker and closed the window so the movie wouldn't be a distraction. Our common interests in mathematics and the sciences were striking. For me, it was particularly fascinating to learn about the emerging field of computer science, the work Ken had been doing at Argonne National Laboratory, and his new job working with the Iliac computer at the U of I. It was my turn to ply Ken with questions. As this conversation moved along, we both marveled at the ease with which we could communicate. We were quickly and increasingly attracted to one another.

On our third date, the next weekend, Ken invited me to a theatrical performance of Shakespeare's comedy, "A Midsummer Night's Dream" and to a very nice restaurant for dinner. When Jan heard what Ken had lined up for that date, she sensed that something important was brewing. She was uneasy with the rapid development of our relationship, especially knowing that Ken was quite a bit older than I. It wasn't that she disapproved, but she simply wondered if it was all going too fast and whether it might interfere with my plans to finish a college degree. As for me that night, I was more preoccupied with what I had available to wear and whether it would be appropriate for the occasion. I had never been to a professional theatrical production, nor to a really formal restaurant before. Fortunately Ken recognized my nervousness and quickly put me more at ease with a smile and a encouraging compliment on my outfit.

We enjoyed the play and the dinner. After dinner, Ken began speaking to me very earnestly. He told me that even though we hadn't known each other very long, he loved me deeply. Then, reflecting his own appreciation of English literature, he cited several lines from Elizabeth Barrett Browning's poem that begins,

"How do I love thee, let me count the ways." I don't really remember exactly what he said right after that because I was so taken aback by what was happening that my mind was reeling. However, I snapped back to complete attention again, a few seconds later, when I heard Ken say, kindly but firmly, that if I was willing, he intended to marry me!

I don't think Ken actually expected me to give him a definite answer right then and there, but rather he wanted to make very sure I knew his feelings and intentions. As I think about it now, he probably had an additional motive. As I learned later (through board games and the way he handled our finances), Ken was a consummate strategist. He knew that I was occasionally dating two men I had met in the James Scholars program who were my own age and not physically disabled. I think he simply wanted to eliminate any possibility of serious competition as soon as possible.

I was very moved and honored by Ken's proposal. I respected him deeply, and there was no doubt that I loved him and that love was growing rapidly, but I also knew that we needed more time to get to know each other better, and I needed to think more seriously about whether I even wanted to be married. I had observed too much pain and strife in my parents' and other marriages to take this step lightly. So I told Ken that I was very grateful for this proposal, assured him that I did love him, but also told him I would need more time before I could give him a definite answer. Out of my deep respect for him, I also promised that while we were considering this step, I would not date anyone else.

After that, we started dating two or three times a week, sometimes going out for special events, but often just having date/study nights, either at the library or sometimes at the office he shared with other graduate assistants in the computer building. Both of us remained seriously committed to doing well in classes, so these dates enabled us to at least be together while we were doing that work. They also enabled us to see each other in different and more realistic situations, uncovering potential areas of conflict and revealing each other's faults.

During this time, I continued to weigh the pros and cons of marrying Ken. On the positive side, Ken simply continued to impress the socks off of me. At age thirty, he was mature, very stable, and strong. He was obviously incredibly capable. He was seeking a PhD in an new and important field. He had already worked two years at Argonne and had a solid job waiting for him there when he finished at the U of I. His analytical mind, the breadth of his interests, and his grasp of history, economics, politics, and current events were also very impressive. He was definitely someone I could love and respect very deeply for the rest of my life. On top of that, he also had a quick and sometimes quirky sense of humor that I secretly adored. Sometimes Ken would make a clever comment or pun with an absolutely straight face, and it might take me up to a half a day to finally get it. When I did, I let him know and we would laugh together—about the pun *and* my slow information processing.

On the negative side, Ken could get very impatient and had a quick temper. However, he also acknowledged these shortcomings, apologized when appropriate, and strove to keep them under control. My most significant reservation, something Ken couldn't help, was his physical disability. It wasn't as though I was prejudiced against marrying someone who was disabled—my own struggle with polio had taught me that a person's real worth and potential are not based on his or her outward physical appearance. My more urgent questions concerned how we would manage if we were to get into difficult situations that neither of us could handle physically or if I would be able to cope with the physical challenges of bearing and caring for children without an able-bodied husband to occasionally step into the gap to assist.

There were a lot of "what ifs" that could have caused us to draw back from marriage. However, both of us had already faced and overcome some very difficult obstacles, and we realized that many others lay ahead of us whether we were married or single. That being the case, it might actually be to our advantage to face those difficulties together so we could work on them as a team. I think my decision in this matter was ultimately influenced more by my heart than by my head. However, as a Christ follower, Ken had the deep assurance that our marriage was in God's will. And since this was so, he was also confident that God would continue to help us every step of the way.

Ken had another quality that was difficult for me to label at the time but which played a critical role in my decision to marry him. He had a certain goodness and kindness in himself that I hadn't observed in any other man. I knew that he was a dedicated Christian. As I thought about this, I became convicted about my own life and wondered whether Ken would still love me and want to marry me if he knew some of the wrong things I had done. Before our relationship went any further, I needed to tell Ken everything that might cause him offense and see if he still felt the same way about me. The thought of doing this made me very anxious because, for all I knew, these revelations could destroy our relationship. Yet if that were to happen, far better that it happen at this stage rather than after we were married.

So I waited for an opportune time and stated that I needed to tell him some bad things about my past. He simply smiled kindly, put his arm around my shoulders, and encouraged me to go ahead and tell him. I was really nervous, but I told him everything and was crying when I finished. When I looked up into his face, he was smiling and had tears in his own eyes. He said, very kindly and lovingly, "Is that all that you were worried about? I could have fallen into any of the same sins in the same situation. All that kept me out of trouble was my lack of opportunity." He went on to share some of the things in his own life that he thought I should know, and that was the end of that conversation. The knowledge that I was completely acceptable to Ken, in spite of my past failures, put my fears to rest and, even more importantly, laid a foundation that later helped me understand how a Holy God could also forgive my sins and accept me unconditionally through my faith in Jesus Christ.

The more I got to know Ken, the more I loved him and wanted to spend my life with him, so it didn't take me long to make a decision. I accepted his proposal at the beginning of November, and we started planning for our future. We both wanted to continue at the U of I, but I discovered that I would lose most of my funding if I got married. Ken wanted to make sure I finished my bachelor's degree, but neither of us wanted to delay marriage two years. Ken came up with a generous and workable solution. He would pay for the rest of my education himself! He had quite a bit of money he had already saved, and he could replenish that supply by working at Argonne during the summers. With that issue settled, we set our wedding date for early June and informed our families.

My family heard the news before they met Ken, and their responses were less than enthusiastic. A few were fully supportive, many gave muted affirmation, but Mom and Orin had serious doubts. Ken's disability was the sticking point. In our rural community, virtually all of my male relatives depended heavily upon their physical strength to earn a living. Consequently, it was very difficult for them to imagine how someone who had to use braces and crutches to walk could possibly provide for himself, a disabled wife, and even children.

Ken received a more encouraging response from his own family, in part because they had a chance to meet me before the announcement, but even more importantly, because they already knew what Ken could accomplish. They had watched him overcome the devastating effects of polio, persevere against incredible odds to get an education, and land a position at Argonne, so they didn't doubt that he could also support a wife and family. Ken's father, Emil, was not so sure about me at first, but Elsie was completely welcoming and affirming. And looking back, this was surprising for several reasons.

Because Elsie's relationship with Emil was strained and because she and Ken had gone through so many trials and victories together, their relationship was very close. She could have quite naturally felt some jealousy toward me or protective toward Ken and discouraged our relationship for those reasons. In addition, both Elsie and Ken were very much aware of the biblical warning that Christians should not marry nonbelievers, and they knew from their own experiences with Emil that such relationships could cause incredible pain. One of Ken's friends even approached him, exhorting him not to take this step. Nevertheless, Elsie remained completely supportive, right from the first.

Sometime after fully committing to Christ myself, I learned about the biblical warning that believers should not marry nonbelievers and immediately asked Ken why he had persisted and married me anyway. Ken told me that he and Elsie had taken this warning seriously and prayed about it at length. However, they stayed the course because both were convinced that Ken had received special instruction from the Lord, and that was what they should trust. As I thought about Elsie's support, I realized that what I was seeing in her was the same kind of love that was shown by Jesus when He died on the cross to pay for our sins. It was an unselfish love that sought the best for Ken and me regardless of its personal cost to her.

That fall, over the Thanksgiving break, Ken and I traveled to Chicago so I could meet his family and visit his home. For a girl from the country who thought Champaign-Urbana was large, seeing Chicago was really an eye-opening experience. When we finally made our way through city traffic and arrived at our destination, I watched with a sense of wonder as Ken squeezed his car into an impossibly small parking space and then climbed the stairs to his parents' apartment. I was a little uncomfortable when I met Emil; however, Elsie quickly put me at ease.

Ken had arranged for me to stay overnight with his aunt and uncle, Judy and Al, in their well-appointed and more spacious house a couple of miles away. Both Judy and Al made me feel welcome, although I had the feeling I was being scrutinized pretty closely by Ken's Aunt Judy, who was probably just trying to make sure I would be a suitable wife. Al, who had been informed about my less-than-prosperous, small-farm background, was immediately accepting, because he had been raised in a very similar circumstances on a farm in Michigan.

On semester break that December, Ken drove to Chicago to be with his family on Christmas Eve and then drove from Chicago to Barry on Christmas Day to be with me and meet my relatives. That evening, when we were alone, Ken gave me a beautiful diamond engagement ring. My first response was astonishment and joy, but inexplicably, that was rapidly overtaken by a growing sense of panic. The ring suddenly made me realize, very concretely, what we were committing to. Troubling questions again raced through my mind. "What if we weren't really compatible or couldn't cope with our disabilities? Would marriage halt my education and deny me a career?" Ken quickly sensed the sudden change in my demeanor and asked what was wrong. I blurted out, in tears, that I didn't know if I could marry him, that I was beginning to change my mind. I even removed that beautiful ring from my finger and gestured that I was giving it back!

Ken was deeply hurt, perplexed, and exasperated by my apparent indecisiveness. He was getting angry and so was I, and we started to argue. Fortunately, before that went very far, Ken recognized that I was being very emotional and regained his own composure. He started asking me questions that forced me to return to more rational thinking. As we reviewed the objective reasons we had agreed upon for getting married, I also calmed down and was reassured that our decision was sound. I felt very foolish for letting my emotionalism tarnish what should have been a completely joyous occasion, but I also came away from that experience with an even deeper confidence in this man who would soon be my husband.

Like it had been for me when I visited Chicago, Ken experienced a bit of culture shock when he visited our farmhouse (which was still without a phone or indoor plumbing). The visit was pleasant though because Ken quite quickly connected with my mother, genuinely enjoyed the meal she had prepared, and made sure to tell her so afterward. He hit it off with Orin right away because of his eagerness to learn more about the farm. They had a lot they could talk about. At that time, I also had three younger siblings at home, all under the age of six, and Ken had a great time playing and joking around with them. He brought his camera with him and made sure to take pictures of everyone so he could share these with Elsie.

During our stay, we also visited other relatives who lived nearby. These visits went pretty smoothly in spite of Ken's physical issues. At that time, his arms and shoulders were so strong that he could get in and out of houses and in and out of chairs using his braces and crutches with remarkably little fuss, and everyone who met him was impressed with his self-confidence and his ability to do these things. Here was a man who was quite capable doing a lot of things they wouldn't even have thought possible. By the time we left, Ken was well accepted, and so was the idea of our marriage. When we returned to campus, we both settled down to study and started planning for our wedding.

Chapter 6

And Then We Were Five

The spring semester before our wedding was a blend of excitement, anticipation, unrelenting busyness, and quite a bit of stress, primarily because we underestimated the amount of time it would take to prepare for our wedding and our new life together. Ken also wanted to maximize the number of days he could work at Argonne that summer, so we set our wedding date for early June, just a few days after final exams.

The first unexpected responsibility surfaced very early in the spring semester when Ken asked me if I had a driver's license. Unfortunately, I did not. I had taken driver's education in my sophomore year but was involved in an accident while driving our family car with a learner's permit. The car was not equipped with turn signals (which were not required at that time), it was dark, and I needed to make a left turn into our country lane. The driver behind me didn't see my hand signal and tried to pass on my left just as I was turning left. There was a fair amount of damage to both cars, but no one was injured. The other driver was at fault, and Mom, who was with me, corroborated that fact, but Orin never trusted me to drive after that. The fright caused by the accident and Orin's continuing distrust badly undermined my confidence. And before I could resume driving and get my license, polio intervened.

After explaining this to Ken, I was about to conclude that I couldn't drive because of the weaknesses in my legs when I realized that this excuse was not going to work. Ken was able to drive quite competently without using his legs at all! His car had an automatic transmission and was equipped with hand controls that allowed him to operate the brakes and the accelerator with his left hand, and to steer with his right hand using a sturdy spinner attached to the steering wheel. Ken assured me that I could easily drive with the hand controls and urged me to get my license as soon as possible. I could get a new learner's permit locally, practice with his car, take the driver's test, and have my license before we were married. When old fears began to surface, I hesitated, but Ken would not let me go there. He insisted that I conquer my fears and move forward!

To encourage me, Ken described his own battle with fear while learning to drive. He hadn't needed to drive before he had polio because he could always use public transportation or his bicycle to get around Chicago. However, when he started work at Argonne in 1957, he purchased a car, had it equipped with hand controls, and asked Emil to teach him to drive. Emil was not very patient, so as soon as Ken had mastered some of the basics in low traffic areas, Emil directed him right onto the Outer Drive along the shore of Lake Michigan and into heavy traffic. When Ken realized where they were headed, he nearly panicked. However, he was determined not to let his dad see that he was afraid, so he focused intently on his driving, managed to avoid accidents, and learned to navigate in traffic in a big hurry. (He also noted, wryly, that this was comparable to learning how to swim by being pushed into the deep end of a swimming pool!) Ken's story left me with no excuse, so I took his advice and, with his encouragement and coaching, obtained my own license about a month before our wedding.

Another task that had to be completed before the wedding was to get our mandatory blood tests and deliver the results, in person, to the courthouse in Pittsfield, Illinois. To save time, we decided to drive there and back in one day—a round trip of 320 miles. The courthouse was not open on weekends, so we chose a weekday that would minimize the number of classes and other obligations we would miss.

That day, Ken picked me up early, and we made our way to Pittsfield in good time. However, right before entering the courthouse, when I checked to make sure I had everything, I discovered that I had forgotten to bring my test results! I was totally exasperated, but there was simply nothing else we could do but drive all the way back to Champaign-Urbana, pick up those results, and make the same trip all over again.

Ken, who had a phenomenal memory, simply could not comprehend how I could forget the very thing we had driven clear across the state to deliver. He was very frustrated and became angry, even asking me if I had left those results behind on purpose! He had every right to be angry, and I apologized with genuine contrition. He accepted that apology, but it took a while for his anger to subside. Fortunately for me, Ken had seen examples of my chronic forgetfulness before, so he finally realized that I wasn't just pulling some kind of cruel joke on him. The trip back was quiet, with both of us contemplating what this incident might be telling us about our compatibility. We did repeat the trip to Pittsfield a few days later, but unfortunately, that day I missed a pop quiz that I could not make up, so I paid a price for my memory lapse!

Another requirement we hadn't anticipated was premarital counseling. We were getting married in my former church in Barry, and the officiating minister believed the counseling was very important. Formal counseling of this type was fairly new at the time, and both Ken and I were a little skeptical, but we agreed to the pastor's request. Pastor Morris asked us to take a marriage compatibility test, which was based upon the assumption that the more beliefs and life experiences a man and woman have in common before marriage, the more likely they were to be compatible and stay married.

We filled out this questionnaire separately. When the pastor compared our answers, however, so many were dissimilar that we literally flunked the test! Ken was from an urban setting, I was from a rural one. Ken was older than me by eleven years and had much more education, and he was a Christian and I was not. The test didn't ask the questions that reflected the important commonalities that we did have, nor could it possibly have predicted the crucial areas of agreement that we would share in the near future, when I, too, fully committed my life to Christ.

Fortunately, Pastor Morris had interviewed both of us before we took this test and was convinced in his own mind that we would be a good match. So he simply acknowledged that such tests can be fallible and continued with the counseling. Ken and I were somewhat disturbed by the results, but they didn't change our plans.

One final item that I needed to attend to was purchasing a wedding dress. We planned to pay for this ourselves to spare my parents this expense. As it turned out, it was fairly late in May when I finally had time to go shopping. Fortunately, without a lot of searching, I found a white satin and chiffon prom dress that was deeply discounted because prom season had recently passed. The dress fit me perfectly, and the length was right, falling at mid-calf. I didn't want a full-length dress because that seemed too formal for our setting, and more importantly, a full-length dress would significantly increase my risk of tripping and falling when I tried to walk in it. I also purchased some additional fabric and other materials from which to fashion a simple veil. Ken was quite surprised and pleased that the total cost for my wedding outfit was less than twenty dollars.

Our wedding was simple and low budget, but it was made memorable and beautiful by the loving generosity, hard work, and ingenuity of my mother, grandmother, and two great aunts. My mother made our wedding cake, a three-tiered beauty, each layer skillfully and artistically decorated, the top layer crowned with a miniature bride and groom. My great aunts both loved flowers and had many in bloom in their gardens at that time in June. They used large numbers of those precious blossoms to make lovely flower arrangements for the church.

I was a little nervous about the ceremony, thinking of all the things that might go wrong. The aisles in the old church were narrow and sloped downward toward the front. Walking down a slope was more risky for both of us than walking on a level floor. What if one or the other of us tripped and fell? My stepfather, Orin, was going to escort me down the aisle, and I knew that holding onto his arm would minimize my risk. However, I couldn't hold onto Ken's arm for support going back up the slope for the recessional. Would I be able to walk back up the aisle without additional support, or would I need to use my clunky metal crutch? Orin was also a very large man, and my dress had one of those very full, bouffant skirts fashionable in the late 1950s and early 60s. What if we would not fit comfortably side by side in the narrow aisles as we marched down to the front of the church?

In spite of my initial misgivings, the ceremony actually proceeded smoothly. Orin escorted me down the aisle without any problem, and Ken and I repeated our vows with deep conviction. We walked single file up the sloping aisle, but finished side by side once we reached the wider, level aisle at the back of the church. I had a large extended family in the area, and my parents had a number of friends and acquaintances who were invited, so our wedding was well attended. Ken's mom and dad and his Aunt Judy and Uncle Al were also there. Our reception, held in an adjoining room, featured the wedding cake, homemade punch, and many other delectable treats prepared by my grandmother and my aunts.

We hadn't planned for a honeymoon because Ken had arranged to start working at Argonne a couple of days after the wedding. Consequently, that first night, we simply stayed overnight in a nearby motel and started off for the Chicago area the next day. Our plan was to live in a furnished apartment in Lombard for three months before returning to U of I.

That night was wonderful, but the next day was full of challenges. About two thirds of the way to Lombard, Ken started feeling ill. By the time we arrived at the apartment, he had a fever and was very sick at his stomach, so he had to lay down and rest almost immediately. I unloaded the things we had packed in the back seat of the car, but when I tried to open the trunk, I discovered that the lock was jammed. Neither keys nor anything else would open it. Ken was too sick to help but told me I needed to find a Plymouth dealership in the phone book, call for an appointment as soon as possible, and take the car in to get the lock fixed.

That would have been very easy for me to do just a couple of months later, but at the time I had not had a lot of driving experience, either with the hand controls or driving in highly congested urban areas. This, plus the thought of searching for a dealership in an unfamiliar area, alone and in heavy traffic, made me very nervous. So on that second day of our married life, at our brand-new apartment, I faced my first significant challenge. I was fearful about driving alone, but I needed to get our belongings out of the trunk before we could settle in for the night. I finally decided that I really didn't have a choice, so I called for an appointment and did make it safely to a dealership for repairs late that afternoon.

Ironically, finding the dealership turned out to be quite a bit easier than getting that trunk opened. The mechanic could not unjam the lock from the outside and realized that he would have to work on it from inside the trunk. To get there, he had to pull out the back seat and remove all of the luggage, books, cooking utensils and other household items that were in the trunk from inside the car. Accomplishing that, unjamming the lock, replacing the seat, and then packing everything back into the car was quite a lengthy process.

When I finally returned to the apartment, Ken was asleep and I didn't want to awaken him. So, I simply unloaded all of our things from the car myself, figured out a way to get all this stuff up the two steps and into the apartment, and then put a lot of it away without disturbing my husband. I was tired when I finished but was encouraged that I had been able to do all this successfully. However, as I thought about all that had happened that day, I couldn't help but wonder what new challenges might lie ahead of us.

Ken recovered from his illness fairly quickly and was able to go to work on schedule. While he was gone, I busied myself organizing the apartment and studying a new Betty Crocker cookbook so I could plan nutritious meals and stock our tiny kitchen with the basics. The next challenge was to see if I could manage the grocery shopping. I hadn't shopped extensively in a large supermarket before, and I didn't know if I could walk through the entire store pushing a loaded grocery cart. Fortunately, this venture also went well. The cart gave me a little extra support when I walked, and it was easy to push. I had help loading the groceries into the car and had already learned how to get bulky items up the steps and into the apartment. My only real challenge that day had been finding all the items on my grocery list.

Ken and I really enjoyed being together, and as we adjusted to married life and learned how to manage the physical obstacles in our new situation, life settled down to a pleasant routine. However, after a few weeks, I started feeling very tired and then sick at my stomach. Ken took me to a doctor to get this checked out. To my astonishment, the doctor told me that I was not ill—I was pregnant! This really caught me off guard. It simply had not registered in my mind that I could actually become a mother, and especially not that fast. That just didn't fit in with our plans!

When I shared this information with Ken, he was less surprised than I had been and genuinely welcomed the news, although he muted his response when he saw my distress. I think he suspected that I might be pregnant from my symptoms and had already been thinking ahead about what we needed to do. However, I was really upset. It was not that I didn't want to have a baby but simply that having one right now really messed up my plans. I didn't want to give up my dream of an education and a professional career. However I still had two years to go before I could even complete a bachelor's degree, and I didn't see how I could continue to attend classes in the latter months of pregnancy or manage schoolwork with the added responsibility of taking care of a newborn. My lingering fear was that if I didn't finish my education right away, I wouldn't be able to get back to it.

Ken was a lot more relaxed about the situation and concluded that we simply needed to settle down, relatively close to Argonne, and he would resume full-time work there to support his growing family. He was concerned about my disappointment, and he remained deeply committed to helping me get all of the education I wanted. However, he also knew from his own experience that one's education could be postponed for a while and resumed later if and when the circumstances warranted.

The doctoral degree Ken was seeking at the U of I really didn't matter that much to him because he was pretty sure that his career would not be affected whether he had it or not. During his two semesters at the U of I, he had taken most of the courses required for that degree, and much of what was left to do was original research. He had already been doing a lot of that at Argonne. For Ken, the knowledge that I was pregnant simply confirmed a strong conviction he already had in his mind. The most important reason that the Lord had guided him to the University of Illinois was not to earn an advanced degree but to meet and marry me!

It took me a while to adjust to the idea of being a mother, and it didn't help that I was fairly ill for many weeks. However, I quickly realized that Ken was right. We needed to find a better place to live and figure out what do about my education later. We also had to act quickly because the lease on our furnished apartment would soon expire. Ken wanted to move to a larger, unfurnished apartment because this would save on rent and give us the extra space we needed.

Thankfully, Ken was able to find an apartment on short notice. It was the first floor of a small house in nearby Villa Park that was reasonably priced and met our most pressing needs. The interior was adequate, but the entrances were problematic. Neither of us could use the front door because it had several concrete steps leading up to it and there was no handrail beside them. There was a wooden stairway up to the back door that did have sturdy handrails, and we could make that work, although it did create some issues. One was how I would be able to transport groceries into the apartment or bring garbage or other items out. Fortunately the landing was fairly large and was level with the back door. And at a height of about three feet, it was low enough for me to set grocery bags or other parcels on it so I could use both hands to get up or down the steps. Once off the steps, I could retrieve what I was carrying and take it to its destination. In addition, the couple renting the second floor of this house were good neighbors and were also willing to help in any way they could.

Once Ken secured the apartment, we needed to purchase furniture and quite a few other household items right away. However, when we started discussing the type of furniture we wanted, we ran into a major roadblock. Suddenly we were disagreeing vigorously and getting into very heated arguments. Consequently, we were both on edge when it was time to go out together and purchase what we needed. Yet in spite of our misgivings, when we saw actual examples of the different styles of furniture, a very surprising thing happened. We found ourselves in almost complete agreement, easily settling on a simple, modern, affordable style known as "Danish Modern."

Shortly after returning home, we set aside time to try to understand why we had had such angry and upsetting arguments before we went shopping. As it turned out, there were two main reasons. Neither of us knew much about furniture styles before we saw examples in the stores, so we were arguing out of ignorance, totally misunderstanding each another. More seriously, both of us were simply determined to have our own way with no thought of compromise! It was humiliating to have to admit it, but we both had a lot to learn about being unselfish and working together as a team.

We needed many other household items and baby equipment, and I found myself really enjoying the day-to-day planning, purchasing, preparing, cooking, and cleaning. I hadn't enjoyed housework much while I was still at home, but setting up and maintaining our own household was a completely different matter. Shortly after moving to the new apartment, my morning sickness also moderated and I truly began looking forward to having our baby.

One big concern about my pregnancy that Ken and I shared was how the weight gain and the shift in the weight distribution in my body in the latter months of pregnancy might affect my balance and my ability to walk and to navigate the back steps. We were particularly concerned about my risk of falling and possibly injuring myself or the baby. Yet even though I climbed up and down those back steps numerous times, I did not fall, and there was always a way and the strength to do whatever I needed to do.

I believe there were three important reasons for this. On the advice of my obstetrician, I kept my weight gain to fifteen pounds. In addition, unexpectedly, my legs, back, and abdominal muscles continued to strengthen significantly during that time even though it had been four years since I had polio. The third and I believe the most important reason was God's continuing provision and protection in response to the earnest prayers of a believing husband and mother-in-law. Thanks to the Lord, I had a healthy pregnancy and a long but normal labor. Our daughter, Diane, was born in the late winter of 1962.

Being a new mom was both exciting and challenging. In this role, I quickly found the fulfillment and sense of purpose I thought I could achieve through an education and a career. It was awesome to look at Diane and to ponder the mystery of how she came to be and how her little body could be formed so perfectly. How could I look at such a wonder and not conclude that there was a Creator? Perhaps Ken's faith in God really did make sense. I didn't act upon those thoughts at the time, but they did make me increasingly receptive to Ken's gentle witness.

Shortly after Diane's birth, Ken and I realized that we needed to move to more accessible quarters. We had both had trouble navigating the back steps, which became hazardous when they iced over repeatedly that winter. They also made it very difficult for me when I had to bring Diane in or out of the apartment. We found a larger and more accessible apartment, not very far away on a quiet street in Lombard, and moved there a couple of months after Diane was born.

Life was much easier there, although Diane developed colic shortly after we moved and would cry inconsolably every evening for several hours. Nothing we could do seemed to comfort her, and even though her pediatrician assured us that this was normal, it was very difficult to bear. Fortunately, that passed in a couple of months. On the other hand, we were both entirely fascinated with Diane's growth and her development of new skills and abilities. During this time, Ken's work was going well and I was growing more confident in my role as a mother and a homemaker. Our larger apartment also made it possible for Elsie to come out on the train from Chicago for occasional weekend visits. She was thrilled to be a grandmother and treasured her time with Diane. She loved to shop for toys and dresses for Diane in her favorite department stores in Chicago.

When Diane was about five months old, I again noticed the telltale signs of morning sickness and our doctor confirmed that I was pregnant again! Both Ken and I were a little shocked at how quickly this had occurred but were also grateful for the good news. By this time, we had experienced the joys of being parents and were much more confident that we could handle the physical demands of parenting. We also had plenty of room in our hearts and our apartment for another child. However, this news, plus the very real possibility that even more children might be coming, did cause Ken to expedite his plans for our future.

Ken didn't want to keep paying rent on larger apartments when he could be applying that money toward purchasing a house. He had never liked the noise and crowding in the center of Chicago where he grew up, and he really didn't care for the suburbs either. I think his long-cherished dream of living in the country was very much on his mind. So was buying property and building a house of his own design. (He had actually spent quite a bit of time studying and designing floor plans as a pastime while convalescing from polio.) Ken also wanted a spacious lot that was fairly private and was graced with large, established trees. So shortly after we learned that our second child was on the way, he told me what he was thinking of doing and we started looking for suitable property.

Ken really liked the area in and around St. Charles, Illinois, near the Fox River, so we began our search there. Before long, we found what he was looking for. The lot was three-quarters of an acre, well drained, and on it there were many very large hickory and oak trees, primarily located around the perimeter of the property. This backdrop created a perfect setting for a house. The property also included one huge old oak tree that a nurseryman later estimated to be at least 300 years old.

Ken purchased that lot in December of 1962, and while he paid it off, he also started working on floor plans. For our projected needs, he designed a simple one-story, three-bedroom ranch with two bathrooms, a standard kitchen, family room, living room, and utility room. For accessibility, he included a large, attached two-car garage that included an indoor ramp into the house. (Having the ramp indoors kept it from becoming slippery in the winter.) Inside the house, he planned for wider than average hallways and doorways to more easily accommodate his wheelchair. Those were the only modifications that we needed at that time.

Our second child, Brian, was born without complications in the early spring of 1963, and our builder started construction on our house in April of 1964. About two and a half months into the house construction, we discovered that I was pregnant yet again! We welcomed the news as before but couldn't help feeling somewhat alarmed, because it seemed like the size of our family was rapidly spinning out of our control. Both of our parents expressed similar concerns, but Ken and I were mainly concerned about how well I could meet the physical challenges of taking care of a three year old, a two year old, and a newborn baby.

Several months later, we learned that we need not have worried about having too many children or about having them too close together. Unbeknownst to us, by the time I gave birth to Niel, in the spring of 1965, I had an advanced case of endometriosis, which prevented any additional pregnancies. In retrospect, once again we could see the Lord's sovereign hand in our situation. If we had been successful in delaying the births of our children, we might never have had them!

By October of 1964, a little over three-and-a-half years into our marriage, we were able to move into our new house with two little children in tow and the third on the way. All this was happening very fast, and we both just continued to marvel at what was taking place. With our children and all of the other changes that just kept coming, we were both continuously facing new physical challenges. But once again, repeating a pattern we had each seen over and over in our lives, there was always a way to do the things that needed to be done and the strength to cope with each new situation. By this point in our lives, thanks to the Lord's consistent provision and guidance, this pattern had become so reliable that we usually didn't question whether or not we could deal with a new physical challenge; we immediately just started praying and thinking about how we were going to meet it.

Ken and I had both come from lower-class socioeconomic backgrounds, so to be in our own home at this early stage of our marriage and to have these beautiful, healthy children seemed a little surreal, particularly to me. Of course, we were only able to make this move so quickly because Ken had entrusted his life to the Lord and had worked right up to his physical limits to get an education and because the Lord had opened doors for him that he couldn't have opened by himself. He was also very frugal and had handled his money wisely from the beginning. His head start on his career at Argonne was also crucial.

Moving day on that early October morning was both exhilarating and exhausting. We hired a mover to pick up and bring out our belongings from the apartment, and both Emil and Elsie drove out from Chicago to give us a hand with putting things away and managing our lively children. The day progressed as smoothly as it could with an eighteen-month old and a two-and-a-half year old running around and getting into things. We all sat down to a meal in the late afternoon, and afterward Elsie and Emil left to drive the fifty miles back into the city. Ken and I busied ourselves putting some more things away and getting Diane and Brian settled in for the night.

It had been a very warm day, and I was determined to take a bath that evening, even though it was late and even though the new light fixtures in the bathroom were not yet hooked up to the electricity. I didn't think that this would be a problem. I could simply turn on the hall light and leave the bathroom door open to get sufficient light. So I filled the tub with warm water and settled back in the semi-darkness to soak.

Ken had gone outside to enjoy the evening (and to celebrate his first night of country living), but after a little while, I heard him coming down the hall in his wheelchair. He peered in and then turned into the bathroom, ostensibly to talk. We did talk for a few minutes, but then I heard something splash softly into the water beside me. A few seconds later, to my horror, I felt that something, which was cool and slippery, move against my legs and realized that

I was sharing the tub with some other living creature! I no idea what it was and no intention of staying around to find out. I scrambled as fast as I could to get up, screaming, "It's alive! It's alive!" and got out of that tub in record time. In the meantime, Ken was nearly doubled over laughing!

He had spotted a good sized toad out in the yard and couldn't resist the thought of putting it in the tub with me, especially since I wouldn't be able to see what it was in the darkness. I have to admit, it took me a while to appreciate his humor because I got very scared and soon after that I got very angry. Nevertheless, it did provide a memorable ending to a very significant day in our lives. And as you probably have guessed, sharing this story with family and friends over the years has generated a lot of laughter.

Homesteading

The first six months in our home were incredibly meaningful and challenging. Shortly after our move, Ken, energized by his new role as a home owner, began thinking about home improvements—specifically about adding some landscaping in front of the house. In addition to shrubs along the foundation, he wanted a low, clipped hedge along the sidewalk that led from the driveway to the front porch. We discussed these ideas and sought advice at a local nursery. The cost of the shrubs was within reason, but the added cost of installation put us over our budget.

Ken was still eager to get this project started, so we explored the possibility of doing some of the planting ourselves. Ken was sure that if he could find a small, short-handled spade, he could do a lot of digging while seated on the ground. At that time, getting out of and back into his wheelchair wasn't a problem because he was able to lower himself to the ground and then raise himself right back into his chair using just his arms and shoulders. I was fairly confident that I could dig with a border spade while standing. Emboldened by all of the new things we had learned we could do, we decided to purchase the shrubs needed for the hedge and plant them ourselves that fall. That way at least the hedge could get off to a faster start in the spring.

We were eager to tackle this project, but it did require a lot more effort than we anticipated. Since the bushes needed to be closely spaced, we basically had to dig a trench that was about two feet wide and deep and twenty feet long. Keeping track of Diane and Brian while we were working on this project definitely slowed our progress, so we were not able to complete it until well into November. By then we were feeling the bite of winter. In fact, a few lazy snowflakes were glittering in the porch light the evening we finally finished.

This project took us close to our physical limits but did teach us some valuable lessons. Working together and using some very unconventional methods, we were able to finish what we started, and that was definitely an accomplishment. However, it was also clear that larger projects like this one should be broken into smaller chunks with plenty of time set aside to complete them—at least while our children were so young.

Another new situation we faced that fall was Ken's long commute to Argonne. When Ken decided to purchase our property, he knew that locating where we did would cost him a daily ninety-mile round trip to Argonne and that he wasn't likely to find other employees nearby with whom he could carpool. However, locating closer to Argonne would have required spending much more money for comparable property and paying significantly higher property taxes. For our family's long-term benefit, Ken deliberately chose to purchase land and build a house that were well within our means and pay the price of the long commute with his own extra time and effort.

Even in the mid-1960s, there was a fair amount of traffic on Ken's route to work, so he requested that we get up at 5:00 am, so he could to be on the road shortly after 6:00. That way he could also leave work early and cut at least half an hour from his commute. I readily agreed because this allowed me to prepare breakfast and spend some uninterrupted time with Ken before our children awoke and my day became very busy.

The distance Ken had to travel and the fact that he was driving alone caused me a lot of concern because I didn't know how he would manage if he had a flat tire or some kind of mechanical breakdown along the way. Ken did not take his wheelchair with him in the car because he used his crutches and braces to get around at work. Consequently, it would have been very difficult for him if he had to get out of the car by the side of the road and try to flag someone down to help. A mobile phone would have solved this problem handily; however, these devices were not yet available.

I was particularly concerned about Ken's safety in the winter. What if he were to slide off in a ditch or get stranded in a snowstorm? It could take quite a while for plows to clear the roads. In those first years, I would watch the clock when it was about time for Ken to return and could get very anxious if he was a few minutes later than normal. However, Ken never seemed to worry about these possibilities. He had prayed repeatedly and earnestly for guidance before purchasing our property, had a clear sense of God's approval, and believed with all of his heart that God would also help him travel safely back and forth to work, so he could provide for his family. (Providentially, Ken was eventually able to locate two other Argonne employees with whom to share at least some of the driving.)

Looking back, Ken's confidence in the Lord's protection was well placed. In all of the trips that he drove by himself during that twenty-five years, he had very few emergencies. (Our mechanical breakdowns and flat tires tended to occur close to or at our home.) I can remember only two such occasions, and in both, the Lord was clearly attending to Ken's safety! In the first incident, Ken was driving home in the dark in a blinding snowstorm and did drive off the road and into a ditch. However, this was actually on our own development road, in sight of our house. Fortunately, a neighbor spotted his stationary headlights, recognized our car, and quickly went out to assist. He helped Ken get out of the car and then brought him the rest of the way home in his own vehicle.

The second incident was even more indicative of the Lord's provision. On that occasion, Ken was driving back from work when his engine suddenly started making strange noises. He quickly pulled the car off the road and stopped, but he didn't have time to get anxious or try to figure out what to do next. Just seconds after he stopped, a pickup truck pulled up right behind him! The driver jumped out, ran up beside the car, and asked if he needed help! Ken, somewhat shaken, replied that he certainly could use help and described what had happened. Oddly, his benefactor didn't seem at all surprised to learn that Ken had to get around on crutches even though this would have been very unusual at that time. Without any awkwardness, he gently helped Ken get safely out of the car and into his own vehicle and then took him to a service station so he could call for a tow and contact me.

Ken saw the man watching and then smiling after Ken nodded to let him know that he was talking with me on the phone, but when he looked back in the man's direction, just moments later, he had vanished and so had his truck! Ken had sensed that there was something unusual about this encounter from the start, and the man's sudden disappearance reinforced that impression. Ken's car had not given any external indications of having problems, so how could this person have known he was in trouble? What were the probabilities that a Good Samaritan would be following so closely behind him on that one rare occasion when he did have car trouble while driving alone? On the trip to the service station, Ken had asked the man his name, but he had countered with a question instead of giving Ken an answer. He also seemed to know that Ken was handicapped, although there were no indications of that on the exterior of the car or the license plates. His sudden disappearance was also puzzling.

Having the mindset of a physical scientist, Ken was always very cautious about assigning supernatural causes to unusual circumstances. He was sure that his swift rescue had been provided by the Lord. However he also came away from that incident with the unshakable impression that his helper was actually an angel! Still, he remained so guarded about this conclusion that he didn't share its more unusual aspects with me until several years after the incident.

Chapter 7: Homesteading

Life in our new home created some challenges too. The house was much larger than our apartment had been, so it required more effort to clean. As our children grew, they also needed more time and supervision. A much more serious concern was related to our children's increasing ability to run. This would not have been a problem for parents with normal physical capabilities, but it could have been for us. At that time, I could walk fairly rapidly but I couldn't run, and I worried about what might happen if one or both of our children decided to run away from me and into danger before I could intervene.

This concern was heightened by an incident that occurred several months earlier, while we were still living in our apartment. Emil and Elsie had given Diane a little red tricycle for her birthday, and that summer she would ride it close to me on the sidewalk by our apartment while I pushed Brian along in a stroller. That particular day, I set the tricycle outside for Diane as usual and stepped back into the apartment to get Brian and the stroller. This didn't take long, but after I got him down the steps and looked around for Diane, she was nowhere to be seen. I walked as fast as I could out to the main sidewalk, past the building next to us, only to see our little daughter pedaling her tricycle away from me, *down the middle of the street*, as fast as she could go!

Diane had a good head start, and I knew I would have a difficult time catching up, so I called out her name and commanded her to stop. She heard me, looked back toward me, and slowed down, but she obviously didn't want to obey. Fortunately, a neighbor was out in her yard, saw what was happening, ran and caught up with Diane, and then carried her and the tricycle back to the safety of the sidewalk. Diane wasn't in too much danger because we were situated on a dead-end street that was mostly used by other tenants. However, this experience was still a wake-up call for me because I could imagine what might have happened if the street were busy or if someone simply didn't see her in time to stop.

Moving to the country decreased that particular risk because our house was a long way from a main road and there was little traffic within the development. However, we did have a very large, unfenced yard with similarly sized undeveloped lots on both sides of our property and farm fields right behind us. Since we were only the third family to build in our subdivision, neighbors were still few and far between. In that situation, I worried that Diane or Brian might run off and get lost in the corn fields behind us. At this age, they were highly mobile but not mature enough to recognize the potential risks of going exploring by themselves. I feared that I would always have to be extra vigilant to keep them from getting into trouble.

However, in retrospect, Diane's escape on her tricycle was the only serious "running-away" incident that either Ken or I encountered. Our children were certainly very active, and they would sometimes run away from me in the house (where I could always catch them), but for some reason, they didn't try to run away from either of us while we were outside or doing shopping. If one or the other started to wander off, a single reprimand would usually bring them back. As I grew more confident of their behavior, I would occasionally take all three shopping with me. I would seat Niel in a shopping cart, and Diane and Brian would walk along beside me. They were usually fairly well behaved and stayed close by on these outings. I have no adequate explanation for this except somehow it was yet another way that the Lord was watching out for us.

It wasn't until I became a grandparent and observed some of our grandchildren's antics that I finally appreciated how remarkable our children's behavior actually was. One grandson, Douglas, loved to run away while his mom was shopping. He would deliberately hide and not respond to her calls so she would have to hunt to find him. When his sister, Rebecca, was not quite three, she decided to take off and go exploring while Diane and I were in our backyard, talking. She deliberately went clear across our yard and directly into a huge backyard in the housing development behind us. She had gotten pretty far away by the time we discovered where she was. Diane tried to call her back, but she just kept on going. Diane actually had to circle around on the development roads in her car to finally catch up with her!

Winter seemed to set in early and decisively right after we finished planting our front hedge. Christmas was not far away, and Ken and I decided to begin celebrating that holiday at our home with Elsie and Emil and our children rather than making the drive to Barry in midwinter, or driving in to Chicago to be with Ken's aunt and uncle on Christmas Eve. We bought a live Christmas tree and thoroughly enjoyed decorating it with newly purchased lights and ornaments. Diane and Brian made Christmas morning lively because they were old enough to get excited about opening presents. That year I also began what would become a fifty-year tradition of preparing Christmas dinner for our family. Elsie and Emil continued to celebrate with Judy and Al on Christmas Eve and drove out from Chicago to be with us on Christmas Day. That first Christmas was particularly meaningful. Ken and I were so blessed to be at this place in our lives, and there was much to be thankful for!

Shortly after Christmas, just a week or so into January, we had several days of freezing rain that quickly built up to record levels. Roads became treacherous, and tree branches and power lines broke under the excessive weight of the ice. Our electric power went off, disabling both our furnace and well pump. We were immediately without heat and would soon be without water. To make matters worse, I was nearly eight months pregnant and definitely feeling the effects of that condition. We hastily bundled Diane and Brian in their snowsuits, put on our own coats, and turned on a battery-powered radio to get more information. The news was not good—the storm damage was very widespread and severe. We would not be getting our electrical power back anytime soon!

The situation was better in Chicago, and Ken's parents still had power, so they invited us to stay with them until our power was restored. I still remember packing, loading the baggage and our children into the car, and watching apprehensively as Ken began the precarious drive to the city. As we paused in our driveway, we could see that many large tree branches were broken and hanging at odd angles or lying on the ground. The tips of single blades of grass that had poked up through the snow had been transformed into large bumps of ice that were one to two inches in diameter!

Our development road and the secondary road leading to the main highway were still coated with ice and were very slippery. As we inched our way along, we could see more tree damage and power lines that were partly suspended and partly lying on the ground. That scene made us both wonder whether moving to the country had really been such a good idea.

As we got closer to town and into more urban areas, the roads were better, so we finished the journey without further difficulty. As it turned out, it was a good thing that we did flee to the city because our power was not restored for seven days and then only with the help of additional crews from Commonwealth Edison that had come in from as far away as Colorado. Fortunately, the weather stayed relatively mild while the power was off, and the water pipes in our house did not freeze and burst. However, our power was restored less than twenty-four hours before a massive cold front moved in. If it had been restored any later, we probably would have had some serious damage to contend with.

After that storm and the disruption it had caused, Ken and I were grateful to get back home and eager for life to return to normal. Since my due date was rapidly approaching, we quickly set to work to finish our preparations for the birth of our third child, equipping the smallest bedroom to serve as a nursery and stocking it with supplies. Unbeknownst to me, while we were preoccupied with that, God was putting the finishing touches on His preparations for my own "New Birth."

During our three-plus years of marriage, I had learned much more about the Christian worldview, primarily from Ken's consistent witness and explanations but also from various pastors and speakers on Christian radio (WMBI) originating from Moody Bible Institute in Chicago. I had learned that God is a God of love but also a God of justice. He created human beings to have a personal relationship with Him, but human sin, rebellion, and disobedience had seriously damaged that relationship. Yet God, in love and mercy, provided another way, through our faith in Jesus and His payment for our sins on the cross, to restore our relationship with Him and to give us eternal life. I also understood that rejecting God's love and rescue plan would lead to eternal separation from God and unimaginable suffering in Hell.

After our move to the country, I began listening to WMBI more frequently, often leaving it on throughout the day while caring for the children and doing my housework. During the first week in February, Moody Bible Institute always hosted a conference called "Founder's Week," and WMBI would broadcast the speakers' messages live. That February in 1965, the speakers seemed to focus on our urgent need to accept Jesus Christ as Savior and Lord and how that could be done. I listened to one convicting message after another, and finally, while sitting at my ironing board, I simply bowed my head and asked God to forgive me for my doubts, pride, stubborn resistance, and other sins, surrendering my life and will to Him entirely. I instantly experienced a very deep sense of peace and freedom and knew immediately that I had made the right choice. By God's grace, from that point forward, I never looked back.

After making this decision, it was difficult for me to understand why it had taken me so long, especially in light of the undeniable and rapidly accumulating evidence that God had been working profoundly in both of our lives. It was as though I was completely discounting what God had done in the past seven years: enabling me to have a strong recovery from polio, providing an open door and the funding for a college education, bringing Ken and me together at the U of I, enabling us to have children, giving us the financial means and enough physical capability to function as responsible parents, enabling us to own our own home, and so much more.

When Ken came home from work that evening, I told him that I had truly repented and given my life to the Lord. He was somewhat cautious at first and asked me a few questions to make sure my decision was genuine and then took me in his arms and hugged and kissed me with great joy, no doubt also thinking back to the powerful assurance God had given him after we had first met that he should marry me and ahead to the immensely positive implications this had for our marriage and our children. As soon as he could, Ken also called Elsie to share with her the good news that I had fully committed my life to Jesus.

The final significant event in that first six months in our home was the birth of our second son, Niel, in early March. Our trip to the hospital was uneventful, delivery progressed normally, and Niel arrived at a healthy eight-and-a-half pounds. The only real challenge that surfaced at that time was the difficulty Ken encountered while taking care of Diane and Brian by himself for the three days I was in the hospital. Elsie took care of Diane and Brian for us while I was in labor, but she had to get back to work the next day.

Ken had already taken a few days off from work to help me with the transition to home, and he didn't think it would be too much of a problem to look after the children himself. Diane was three and Brian was nearly two, so both of them could walk wherever they needed to go. Diane was pretty well potty trained, but Brian was still in diapers. Ken had helped me with bathing, dressing, feeding, and diapering on a number of occasions, and he could easily catch and pick up the children while in his wheelchair. I had also prepared frozen meals that he could simply pop into the oven and warm so everyone would have good food to eat.

What Ken didn't anticipate was the challenge of keeping track of both the kids for extended periods of time, making sure they didn't get into mischief, and trying to juggle priorities when they both needed his help at the same time. When I talked with him by phone that first day, Ken was not very happy. Apparently Diane and Brian had been more mischievous than usual and Diane had regressed with the potty training. He had spent a lot of time just trying to clean up their messes. He tried not to complain, but I could tell that he was having a very difficult time managing all these issues from his wheelchair.

Ken was visibly relieved to bring me home from the hospital so life could start returning to normal, even though I was bringing a newborn with me to add to the mix. He told me afterward that taking care of Diane and Brian by himself was one of the most difficult things he had ever attempted! For someone who had overcome and accomplished so much, that was a very significant statement! This experience definitely increased his appreciation for the daily work I was doing at home.

This period when our children were all very young provided us with many fond and funny memories. One the most unforgettable was watching Diane's and Brian's reactions to Niel when they first had a good chance to look at him after we brought him home from the hospital. I had taken him into the room we were using as a nursery and had laid him in a low portable crib that had nylon netting on all sides. When we told them to come in and see their new brother, Diane and Brian solemnly entered, hand in hand, and walked side by side to the crib, pressing their little faces tight against the netting to get a closer look. They remained in that same position for a long time and were unusually quiet, perhaps because Niel was asleep, but we could tell that they were very intrigued. This was just the first of many and much more lively visits they would make to see and interact with their new sibling.

A few months after Niel was born, Ken and I began discussing our need to find a church where we could attend regularly and involve our children. While living in the suburbs, we occasionally visited Emanuel Covenant, Ken's home church in Chicago, and two other churches not far from where we lived, but after our move, these were all more than twenty-five miles away. To be actively involved, we needed to find a church close by.

Ken started making inquiries and learned from one of his friends at Emmanuel that there was a small Evangelical Covenant church, Lily Lake Church, just seven miles from our home. Ken was immediately intrigued. He was comfortable with Covenant doctrine and was attracted by this denomination's connection to his Swedish heritage. (The Evangelical Covenant Church had split off from the Swedish Lutheran Church in Sweden, so Covenant churches in this country typically had congregations that included quite a few Swedish descendants.) Moreover, some of the members at Emmanuel knew members at the Lily Lake Church.

Since the church was so close, we immediately drove by to check it out and see whether it was physically accessible. Ken was immediately captivated by its simple country charm—its plain white rectangular shape and the prominent steeple above the front entrance. The church appealed to me because it was small and members would likely know each other well. The front entrance had several steps, so we could see that getting in would not be easy. However, it was possible because it also had a sturdy handrail.

We didn't try to attend the Lily Lake Church until Niel was about two and fully mobile, because I would not have been able to carry him up the steps. We also wondered whether our obvious physical disabilities would adversely affect how members at the church would accept us. I could climb the steps in a fairly ordinary way using my short crutch and the handrail; however, Ken's manner of navigating steps and getting in and out of pews was definitely unusual and would undoubtedly attract a lot of attention, especially in a small congregation among people we did not know.

The Sunday we decided to visit, we hustled to get ourselves and all three children dressed in their Sunday best, drove to the church, plucked up our courage, and made our grand entrance, trying to be as inconspicuous as possible. To our surprise and relief, Ken and I and our little troupe were greeted warmly and were well accepted from the start. This became our home church for many years.

The first year we attended, the church didn't have a separate nursery or preschool area, which meant that children had to sit with their parents and behave. This usually worked out fairly well for us except for one Sunday when our pastor was ending the service with a long prayer after a very long sermon. Niel started fidgeting, and we struggled to keep him quiet. To our surprise (and horrified amusement), he started saying, "Amen." At first he said it rather softly, but then he started repeating it, getting louder each time. Diane and Brian knew he was doing something wrong and watched uneasily to see what we would do. Some of the older children and adults sitting close to us also heard Niel and struggled to stifle their laughter. We eventually got Niel to stop, but not before he had repeated "Amen" several times.

We were sitting close to the back of the church, so I do not know whether our pastor actually heard Niel or just noticed some unusual restlessness and stirring in the congregation, but it wasn't long before he said, "Amen," himself. No harm was done, and we laughed every time we recalled this episode. However, neither of us ever figured out how our very young son came up with this particular word and insisted upon repeating it right at the proper but potentially most embarrassing part of the service!

Chapter 8

Growing Together

Our first few years in our home were filled with new challenges and opportunities. Now that we had settled into a permanent location, adapted to family life, and were in agreement on our faith, Ken and I began thinking more intentionally about our goals as parents. Our first priority was to help our children come to saving faith themselves, through our example, instruction, and active participation in a church. We wanted them to be involved in Sunday school and youth activities and grow up with like-minded friends. Ken was especially resolute on this latter point because he had been very positively influenced in his own faith by his experiences in Christian camps and in the friendships he had developed with other young people at his church. We also committed to praying consistently that each of our children would eventually accept Jesus as his or her own personal Savior and Lord.

Another very strong priority we shared was to provide a secure, loving, and peaceful home. Both of us had grown up with broken relationships, arguing, instability, and bitter conflict in our own families, and we wanted no more of that. However, after four years of marriage and the addition of three children, we also realized that wanting peace and stability in one's family and actually achieving it could be two different things. Marriage, with its demands that two people learn to share, compromise, and submit to one another consistently, helped us begin to see just how selfish, stubborn, and quick to retaliate we both could be. Trying to meet all the needs of our small children periodically exposed these and other faults even more clearly. Our growing appreciation of the basic sinfulness of human nature was strengthened further when we observed how early these same traits appeared in our children. Sinful behavior was obviously something they didn't have to learn!

This recognition of our own weaknesses along with the Bible's clear teaching on the subject made it obvious that we could not achieve the peace and stability we desired in our own strength. We needed to be honest about our failures with each other and ask for God's forgiveness and help in this endeavor. Just like our children, we needed to keep on growing. As they grew into physical maturity, we needed to be growing into spiritual maturity—in our relationship with each other, with them, and with God.

Ken and I had both learned the value of hard work and self-discipline, and we definitely wanted to help our children learn to value these attributes as well. As a consequence, we started training them to help with smaller chores as soon as they were able (such as picking up and putting away their toys, putting dirty clothes into the laundry basket, and so on). As they grew, we gave them increasingly more challenging responsibilities. We also tried to avoid getting into heated arguments in front of the children, waiting until they were not around or going into our bedroom and shutting the door to settle these disputes privately. Fortunately, taking this precaution wasn't necessary very often.

In addition to setting some parental goals that first spring, we also had some new-home-owner responsibilities to attend to. The grass in our very large yard had begun to grow and would soon need to be cut. Ken wanted to do this job himself and was confident he could do so if he could find the right equipment. After some research and shopping around, we found a rider mower equipped with controls that didn't require the use of one's legs or feet. Once the mower was delivered, Ken had to figure out a way to get from his wheelchair onto the mower. He had to try several different approaches, but he finally discovered a two-step process that worked. He first lifted himself from the wheelchair onto the mower fender and from the fender to the mower seat. He practiced driving for a few minutes and then was ready to mow.

One problem Ken hadn't anticipated was the need to first pick up dead wood and smaller branches that regularly fell to the ground from our trees. I walked around in the yard and did the pickup for a few weeks until I happened to discover a very handy device called a "grabber" in a mail-order catalogue. This was a lightweight pole with a handle and a trigger on one end and a pair of "claws" on the other end that could be used to grab items that were otherwise out of reach (like a can of food on a high shelf, or an object accidentally dropped behind an appliance or heavy piece of furniture). The grabber was sturdy enough for Ken to use to pick up pieces of wood and branches from the ground while seated on the mower. He would stack these behind his legs or on his lap until he had a full load and then drive to the burn pile to drop them off. Using this technique, Ken was able to do the mowing each week pretty much by himself.

While he was mowing, I was usually working inside the house, but I would listen for the sound of the mower and occasionally check his progress visually through a window. If the motor stopped and for some reason he couldn't restart it, he would be stranded in place until I could bring him his wheelchair. If the mower malfunctioned, Ken would drive it into the garage and I would hear him and come out to assist. He would transfer from the mower to his wheelchair and then to the garage floor, if necessary, to make repairs. Poring over the manual and working together, we could usually find a way to troubleshoot and fix the problems.

After that first mowing season, Ken was confident that he could handle this job. That helped persuade him to purchase the lot adjacent to the one we already owned. He did this partly as an investment, partly to give us more space and privacy as the development built up around us, and partly because the second lot could be added seamlessly to our existing lawn. That purchase increased the size of our lawn to one-and-a-half acres! Fortunately, we didn't have to do anything to that lot except an initial cleanup. The sturdy and self-sustaining mix of bluegrass and white clover that was growing there only needed to be cut regularly. After mowing it for a year or so, the long, unbroken expanse of bright green grass and stately trees across the back of both lots made our yard look like a park!

The downside of adding the extra land was the additional work this created for Ken. It doubled his mowing time to about three hours every week, but he didn't mind. He enjoyed being outside and doing physical work any time and in any way that he could. I know it was also very gratifying for him just to be outside, enjoying an uncluttered view and the country air, as he had always longed to do while living in Chicago. Incidentally, Ken continued to do the mowing until Brian and then Niel were old enough to do it, and they were assigned that duty as long as they lived at home. However, when they moved away, Ken picked up the job again and was able, by God's amazing provision, to continue doing it until he was seventy-five years old!

While Ken was making the lawn look good that first summer, I was thinking of ways to make the interior of the house more attractive. As always, I was keenly aware that whatever I wanted to do, I needed to stick to our budget. We didn't yet have curtains for some of the windows, so I found some instructions for sewing curtains and drapes, purchased the appropriate hardware and fabrics, and proceeded to sew and hang these myself. I also wanted to change the paint color in one of the children's rooms, so I tried to think of a way that I could paint the room myself. I had found a way to get up and do some things from the second step of our stepladder, but that didn't put me high enough to paint a careful straight edge between the top of the wall and the ceiling.

One thing I had learned to do with some facility was to lower myself safely to the floor (or the ground) from a standing position and then get up again without a chair or anything else to lean on for support. I couldn't just bend my knees, crouch and then raise myself with my legs because of permanent weaknesses in the quadriceps muscles in both legs. However, I did discover that I could start on my hands and knees, gradually straighten my legs, and move into an upside down V with both hands and feet on the floor and the bend at my waist. With both knees locked, I could then use my back and arms to raise the upper part of my body to a fully upright position. (I and my family jokingly referred to this as my "teepee" maneuver.)

As I was thinking about this maneuver, I suddenly realized that I could do this from any flat stable surface that was large enough—it didn't have to just be the floor. I could actually use our large sturdy dining table, covered with a drop cloth, to create a suitable platform from which to paint. All I had to do was move the table into position, sit on the table, get on my hands and knees, and then to my feet. This would put me at a comfortable height to paint the even edge I needed at the ceiling. I could do the edge at the floor while sitting on the floor, and then use a roller with an extension handle while standing to paint the walls. This method did require quite a bit of physical effort and concentration, but it worked. I used it to successfully paint not only that first year but many years thereafter when I wanted to change wall colors.

Finding ways to do tasks like these, which had seemed beyond our physical abilities, became incredibly meaningful to us. We both had to learn new ways of doing many ordinary things after polio, and the need for innovative solutions just kept growing after we married, had children, and then became homeowners. However, time after time, as each new challenge came along, there was also a solution. It became very clear to both of us that the Lord was helping us use the capabilities that we did have to accomplish things we had previously thought impossible. As gratifying as these accomplishments were, the greatest reward, by far, was the evidence they provided of the Lord's ongoing assistance and blessing in our lives.

I don't know if this was a sign of overconfidence, but our successes with mowing and home decorating in the summer of 1966 encouraged us to take on even more demanding home-improvement projects during the next three summers. In the spring of 1967, I decided I wanted to create a small vegetable garden. When this thought first came to me, I was ambivalent because I remembered the long, sweaty hours I had been compelled to spend in our garden on the farm. However my situation was different now, and there were good reasons for reconsidering this option. For one, I did have a strong interest in gardening. The previous fall, a gardening friend had potted up several geraniums that were in full bloom to rescue them from the frost. She gave two of them to me, and I tended these carefully through the winter and watched with great delight as they broke into bloom again in the very early spring. I hadn't realized how rewarding it was to grow flowers.

I also knew that our property had been partly wooded pasture land for at least 100 years, and judging by the age of our trees, it had probably never been seriously farmed. As a result, the soil on our property was very rich. I couldn't help but wonder how the vegetables that grew well in the clay on our farm would produce in the fertile black loam in our yard. I also knew that even a small vegetable garden could produce a lot of food, could save on our food bill, and would probably offer us superior nutrition as well. When I realized that I also had a perfect, sunny area for a garden on our second lot, the issue was settled.

The first garden patch was pretty small, only about eight feet long and wide. However before I could plant, we first had to remove the tough, well-established sod, turn over the soil with a pitchfork, and then break it up with a hoe and a rake, so it took quite a bit of physical effort to prepare even this small area. Ken helped me take up the sod, but I had to do the digging and cultivating because his wheelchair would mire down in the loose soil. I planted several different vegetables and a few flowers in my new garden and was very richly rewarded with the fruits of my labor that first year. After that, Ken was convinced of the garden's value and I was hooked. Gardening became one of my passions. Predictably, that vegetable garden continued to grow larger over the years, much to the sometimes exaggerated dismay of our children when they were asked to help hoe or pull weeds to keep it tended.

That same year we created the garden, Ken decided that we needed to add an extension on one side of our driveway so that we or our visitors could park there without blocking access to the garage. Ken wanted to excavate a space that would accommodate two vehicles side by side (about 500 square feet) and could be filled with eight inches of limestone gravel to connect seamlessly with our existing driveway. When Ken called excavation companies for pricing, he discovered that the cost of this job was more than he wanted to pay, so he decided he would do this job mostly by himself!

Ken first purchased a very sturdy steel cart that could be pulled by the mower to haul away the dirt that needed to be removed. He sat on the ground to do the work, first stripping away the sod and then removing the dirt, one shovel full at a time, using only his arms, shoulders, and back muscles to dig and to throw the dirt into the cart. I helped him a little with the sod removal and digging, but my main task on this project was to haul away the cartloads of dirt with the mower and unload them. (Unloading was relatively easy because cart was equipped with a removable back panel and the bed tilted back so the dirt could slide out by itself.) Ken kept at the digging on weekends and after work, and when he finished, he ordered a truckload of gravel and had it dumped in the excavated area. Ken and I and even Diane and Brian (then five and four) took rakes and shovels and spread this gravel evenly in the space to finish this job.

Early in the spring of 1969, Ken thought of another improvement that he wanted to make. At that time, the north side of our property had very few trees and the land adjacent to it had none, since it had been a farmer's field before the land was developed. Consequently, our house and property were really exposed to winds from the north and the west. Because of this, we would consistently have very large snowdrifts that would form parallel to the front of our house, making it difficult to get in and out of the garage or the front door. (We had to shovel through drifts quite a few times to keep access open.)

For a few years, we put up a snow fence parallel to the driveway to break up this pattern and that helped. However, Ken wanted a more permanent solution. He reasoned that a double row of white pines across the northern and part of the western boundary of our property would form a very effective windbreak. This would minimize the drifting problem, decrease our heating bills, and increase privacy in the yard. Truth be told, Ken also just loved trees and was always looking for a good excuse to plant a few more of them. White pines were his first choice because they were native to our area and he had admired these stately trees in the mountains of Colorado and in the north woods of Wisconsin when he attended camps there as a teenager. He also learned that the US Forestry Service sold evergreen seedlings in large quantities for only pennies apiece and decided that this would be an inexpensive way for us to create the windbreak.

Ken had to buy a bundle of 250 white-pine seedlings to take advantage of this deal, which was about 150 more than we planned to plant, but he found friends and colleagues at work who quite willingly took the extras. When planted, these seedlings were only about three to four inches high, so they didn't require large planting holes, but we did need to remove a larger circle of sod for each hole, and each seedling also needed to be carefully watered in. With 100 seedlings to plant, we knew that this job would take significant time and effort.

Fortunately, I had a good friend who heard about our project, and she graciously volunteered herself and her husband to help. Lena and her husband had two boys who were just a little older than our own children, so they came too and played with our children while the four of us planted all those trees. We shared a picnic lunch around noon on that day and finished the planting in the late afternoon. Those pine trees grew very slowly for the first ten years, and mowing around them was difficult. However, after that, the trees started growing about a foot a year, quickly filling in the space to create the effective and striking windbreak that Ken had envisioned.

In addition to our various home improvement projects, Ken also had a keen interest in traveling, seeing new places, and taking pictures that could later be projected and viewed on a large screen. Ken hadn't had much opportunity to travel until after he started working and owned his own car. After that purchase and before we met, Ken took two long trips with his mother, Elsie, one to the East Coast and up into Canada and the other to the Rocky Mountain states. After we met, married, had children, and then became homeowners, for a while we needed to use all of our resources to meet our rapidly changing needs. Consequently, for several years, we didn't attempt to travel much further than the 280 miles required to visit my family in Barry.

Ken's interests in traveling and seeing new things had not diminished during that time. He was simply biding his time until the children were a little older and our budget would not be strained by the cost of traveling. He was eager to start traveling again, especially so he could share these new experiences with us. In the early spring of 1968, Ken decided that we were finally in a good position to take a long vacation together. This sounded really exciting to me, so we started discussing where we would go and how we going to accomplish this.

Ken was eager for me to see the Rocky Mountains and thought our children, who were then seven, six, and four, would be old enough to enjoy that experience as well. Ken's preference for this trip was to visit some of the spectacular national parks and national monuments located in Colorado, Arizona, and Utah and to follow some scenic drives in the mountains. We decided that we would stay in motels at night, take or purchase food for breakfast and lunch, and eat in restaurants only in the evenings. Another priority was to find motels that offered swimming pools and/or playground equipment that we knew our children would enjoy in the evening. Ken set to work planning a daily itinerary, and I started making lists of the clothing and other gear that we would need. Ken envisioned a three-week trip, starting the last week in May, after Diane was out of school, and extending into the middle of June.

As we set off together in the car that early morning in May, we were all filled with excitement and anticipation. The first few hours of travel went well, but then Diane, Brian, and Niel started getting restless and began to argue and find fault with each other. They had to share the back seat of our full-sized car, but that suddenly didn't provide enough space. The seat cover seams divided the space into three sections, and all three children started getting very territorial. If one accidentally (or intentionally) moved an arm or leg in a way that invaded someone else's space, the offended party would protest immediately. Games, puzzles, coloring books, and occasional reprimands from their dad or from me would tone down the skirmishes for a while, but they would inevitably return. It became clear that we were going to have to make more frequent and longer stops than Ken had planned for if we were going to retain any semblance of peace. This frustrated Ken. Like the precise planner and mathematician that he was, Ken had prepared a careful itinerary, trying to optimize the number of national parks and places of interest we could visit. However, our need to stop more frequently altered those plans on the very first day.

The next two days as we drove across the country to reach the mountains, we faced the same problems. When we finally reached the foothills and began stopping more frequently, our children did become more interested in their surroundings and were able to work off more energy when we did stop. As a result, the back-seat squabbling decreased, but it still did not disappear.

Ken had planned for us to see a number of different places of interest, and because these were quite a few miles apart, most of our motel stays were for a single night. This created another source of irritation that neither of us had anticipated. Traveling this way meant that every morning, in addition to setting out breakfast and getting the kids ready to go, I also had to repack everything and load it into the car before we could leave. That inevitably took more time than Ken had planned for, so he was usually impatient to get started. Of necessity, I had to do most of this work, and I did get more efficient with practice, but I was getting more and more irritated by Ken's consistent impatience because it seemed to be directed at me.

A few days into our trip, and after a particularly frustrating drive through beautiful scenery that we couldn't enjoy very much because of the jostling and arguing going on in the back seat, we were both pretty annoyed. After we unpacked at the motel that night, Ken's patience snapped and so did mine and we got into the most serious argument we had had since getting married. Fortunately, this happened after all three children had gone out to play in the swimming pool, so they didn't hear our angry exchange.

In the midst of our argument, I suddenly remembered that I needed to check on the children, and as I stepped out of our motel room to do so, I was met by Diane, who was very wet, very angry, coughing, and sobbing uncontrollably. It wasn't entirely clear what had actually transpired, but it appeared that Brian and Niel had urged her to jump through an inner tube that they were holding in the deep end of the pool. The jump went badly, she swallowed some pool water, panicked, and then got very angry with her brothers. The incident snapped both of us back to reality when we realized what could have happened. Our angry argument had distracted us from the responsibility of supervising our children while they were in the swimming pool, and the outcome might have been tragic. We needed to identify and deal with the real issues that were bugging us and stop attacking each other.

After the children were in bed and we had time to talk, we both apologized and tried to identify the real reasons for our argument. Ken was disappointed because he had wanted the trip to be a time for us to grow in our relationships and to learn more about God's amazing creation, and this wasn't happening. But he was also irritated because his careful plans had been compromised, impatient because we couldn't seem to stick to a schedule, and felt very frustrated and guilty because he couldn't do the physical work of packing and unpacking the car himself, so all that work necessarily fell to me. I was frustrated because my ability to enjoy and ponder the implications of the grandeur I was seeing was being hindered by the children's poor behavior, because Ken was obviously unhappy, and because I thought that he was irritated with me. As we talked these things through, we both recognized the our fundamental problem was simply that our children were not yet old enough to appreciate the things that were so meaningful to us. We needed to modify our plans, see fewer places, and give the children more time each day to do the things they really enjoyed.

In spite of its difficult beginning, the rest of this vacation was far more relaxed and enjoyable, and we were still able to see and admire many natural wonders. I had not been any further west than eastern Missouri, so I thoroughly enjoyed seeing the different landscapes, trees, plants, and animals along the way. And I was absolutely awestruck when we finally made it to the Rocky

Mountains. I vividly remember our first visit to Rocky Mountain National Park. The grandeur of the mountains was absolutely breathtaking, and just as it had been for Ken the first time he saw them, it was a deeply spiritual experience for me as well. What an awesome God that He would create such majesty and beauty and, in addition, create human beings with the capacity to see, enjoy, and marvel at His handiwork.

One memory that remains especially vivid was a time we stopped in a larger pullout area in Rocky Mountain National Park. After spending some time there getting pictures and admiring the view, I suggested a snack—chocolate chip cookies that I had made at home and hidden away so we could pull them out and enjoy them on just such an occasion. As we were sitting at a picnic table, we saw three little chipmunks timidly approaching our table. (Apparently they liked what they were smelling.) We couldn't resist sharing some little pieces of cookie. The chipmunks, their tiny bodies quivering in anticipation and fear, came very close to us to snatch these pieces away, to the total delight and amazement of our children.

Some other very memorable events from that first trip come to mind as well. Ken was eager to see and snap as many good pictures of the places we were visiting as possible, and this meant that he had to walk out to various lookouts and other points of interest using his crutches and braces. Quite a number of places were just not accessible for Ken, and this was often frustrating. On those occasions, I would go out with the children to look and take some pictures myself.

On this particular day, we were beside a spectacular, roaring mountain stream, and Ken was determined to get a good close-up shot himself. To do so, he had to move dangerously close to the edge of a high drop-off. I was apprehensive as he started this maneuver, and then to my horror I saw one of his crutches start to slip in the loose gravel. Fortunately Ken was able to regain his balance, and then he slowly and carefully backed away to safer ground. If he had not regained his balance, he could have easily fallen right over the edge!

On another occasion we were driving on a fairly narrow, winding mountain road. The day was very warm, and we had the car windows open because we didn't have air conditioning. Suddenly a wind gust swept through the car and Diane's hat, which she loved, went flying out of the car window. Diane was beside herself and begged us to stop and rescue her hat. Unfortunately, we had seen the wind whip it across the road and down the mountainside, so there was no way to retrieve it. She was very unhappy about that loss the rest of the day.

Another time in a similar situation on a mountain road, a very large insect flew in a back window, sending all three children into a full-blown panic. Ken had all he could do to control his laughter at their antics and to concentrate on staying on the road. (Driving on narrow, winding mountain roads was a bit of a challenge using the hand controls.) In spite of my efforts to calm things down, the uproar in the back seat continued until we finally came to a spot where Ken could pull over and I could get out and remove the "ferocious looking" intruder.

When we arrived at home after that first long family trip, we returned with many exciting memories, a cache of excellent pictures, and some valuable life lessons. One of those lessons for Ken and for me was that we shouldn't try any more long, sight-seeing vacations with our children for a few years. While they were young, we took shorter trips that offered plenty for them to do that we were sure they would enjoy.

Chapter 9

Continuing Education

In the earlier years of our marriage, Ken and I were completely occupied with our family, home, his work, and our friendships at church. We were also very grateful that God had given us the physical ability and opportunities to participate fully in all these things. Yet even in the midst of all this fullness, I was gently reminded from time to time that I had still had some unfinished business to attend to. What did I intend to do about continuing my education?

I had signed up for a correspondence course from the University of Illinois shortly after we decided not to return to campus, thinking that I could complete it before Diane was born. However, it wasn't until I was eight months pregnant with Brian that I was finally prepared to take the final exam. After Brian arrived, with our move to St. Charles and Niel's birth shortly after, I simply didn't think seriously about further study until 1966, when our children were four, three, and one. By that time, my values had changed considerably.

Somewhat paradoxically, it was my decision to accept Christ the year before that helped persuade me to continue. Before becoming a Christian, I wanted an education primarily to gain prestige and recognition. After accepting Christ and growing in my faith, those motives seemed worthless, even sinful. What I had actually needed was love, acceptance, and a sense of meaning and purpose in my life. The Lord provided all of these through my roles as a wife, mother, and Christ follower. So if I already had the love, fulfillment, and purpose that I had longed for, was there any good reason to press on for a career? Should I simply concentrate on being a full-time mom and serving in our church?

Ken and I discussed and prayed about this issue at great length. Being a full-time wife and mother would certainly have been the easier route to take, and I could see sound reasons for doing this from Scripture. On the other hand, continuing with my education would require a great deal of time and effort and a lot of help and understanding from my family. Still, I did have a definite sense of calling and knew in my heart that continuing on was something I should do, even though I did not know specifically where that might lead. Both of us also reasoned that God had given me the academic ability I had for a purpose and He probably expected me to develop and use it in some way.

Another factor that we considered was our children's education. Both of us were committed to providing each of them with a college education if they chose to pursue it, which meant that I would eventually need to go to work to help pay for those expenses. Since an interesting, well-salaried job seemed more likely if I had a bachelor's degree, we agreed that this should be my immediate goal. If for some reason that didn't work out, I could always discontinue and nothing would be lost. If my sense of calling was legitimate, the Lord would help me succeed. Whatever the case, it would be far better to try and fail than not to try at all.

It was clear to both of us that if we wanted to safeguard the well-being of our children and the quality of our family life, finishing a bachelor's degree could take a long time. I would start very gradually and try to minimize my time away from home until the children were older. I knew I could take some of needed courses by correspondence. I also discovered that our home was only twenty miles from Northern Illinois University in Dekalb, Illinois.

Providentially, NIU offered a wide selection of night classes for part-time commuter students, which met only once or twice a week. Taking night classes would allow Ken to be at home with the children while I was away at class. The commute would not take too much time because the route to Dekalb ran through open farmland.

Since NIU was the closest four-year institution, it was also the logical place from which to get my bachelor's degree. In the spring of 1966, I switched my major from physics to psychology to pursue a strong interest I had in learning more about the human brain and its relationship to human experience. I compiled a list of courses I would need and then began the long journey to the BA with a correspondence course on Shakespeare from the University of Illinois. After finishing that, a year later, I took my first night class, Speech 101, at NIU. It was exciting to be back on campus and rewarding to be learning a new skill. My enjoyment of this course helped assure me that I was moving in the right direction.

Over the next four years, as the children grew and entered grade school, I gradually added more evening and correspondence classes. Finally, in the fall of 1971, when the children were nine, eight, and six, I tackled the requirement of being a full-time student for a semester and finished the sixteen hours of coursework needed for my degree. It had taken me ten years to complete the requirements that would have taken two years of full-time work on campus. However, during that same ten years, in addition to the BA, I had also earned an MRS and three MOMs, and these were and will always be the most significant and satisfying accomplishments of my life.

Summaries have a way of making difficult endeavors seem simple and straightforward. However, the actual process of getting that degree was arduous, and I certainly could not have done it alone. There were many challenges along the way and many times when I second-guessed my decision to continue. One of the most difficult issues that kept replaying in my mind was whether this undertaking was depriving my children or my husband and whether

I was actually slipping back into the self-focused ambition that drove me before I accepted Christ. This concern led me to pray frequently that the Lord would help me stay entirely within His will. Moreover, I had a *lot* of wholehearted help and encouragement along the way from Ken, who never wavered in his support, and from our own children, Ken's parents, and the Lord Himself.

One thing I learned very quickly from my first class back on campus was that I was going to have to find more time for study if I wanted to take more than one class at a time, so I explored ways of doing housework more efficiently, especially meal preparation. I discovered that I could save a lot of time by preplanning our meals for an entire month and then preparing suitable entrees and casseroles in big batches and freezing meal-sized portions for future use, especially for nights when I would be away. By preplanning, and doing careful inventories, I was also able to cut grocery shopping to once every three or four weeks.

When I discussed my need for more study time with Ken, he suggested that I make a list of all my household chores and then went over this list with me to identify the jobs he or our children could do with reasonable efficiency. To his credit, Ken never faltered nor complained when he had to do extra work or to keep our children on task in this family venture.

One practice we began right away was asking the children to pick up and put away their toys and clothes each evening and on Saturdays so I could clean more efficiently. They also learned to dust the furniture, make their own beds, and help fold clean laundry. I would start the laundry early each Saturday morning, and when everything was clean and dry, we would all gather around the table with the laundry baskets, each of us folding and putting away our own clothes plus some additional items. Neither Ken nor our sons really liked this chore, but they all stuck with it. However, the three of them did consistently engage in a lot of bantering and teasing in the process. I never did figure out whether this was an indirect form of protest or simply a way to relieve their boredom.

One activity that occupied a significant amount of my time on weekdays was fixing lunches for school, especially making sandwiches. When the children were a little older, I tried having them assemble their own sandwiches and lunches, but this was not a good idea because it inevitably created a lot of traffic and turmoil in our small kitchen at the last minute, right before it was time for them to get out the door and catch the school bus.

Always searching for greater efficiency, I hit upon the idea of making the sandwiches in advance, bagging them individually, and then freezing them. That way all we would have to do in the morning was to grab the sandwiches from the freezer. The idea was appealing because sandwich preparation was a task we could do in assembly-line fashion around the table. With a little practice, we were able to prepare the sandwiches needed for two weeks very quickly. However, I had not anticipated the unpleasant effects that freezing and thawing would have on the bread and sandwich ingredients (especially peanut butter and jelly). The kids really did not appreciate their soggy sandwiches, so their sandwich-assembly duty didn't last very long.

Since we did not have a dishwasher, cleaning up the dinner dishes also required a chunk of my time every evening. Ken came up with a scheme to relieve me of that duty—he and our crew would do this for me. Every month he took a page from a calendar and wrote the first letter of either his own or one of the children's names on each day, on a rotating schedule, and posted it in the kitchen. It was the duty of the person signified to wash the dishes that evening. He also made a rule to ensure good quality control. If in his or my judgment, one of the children had more than three items that had not been cleaned satisfactorily, that person would also have to wash the dishes the next evening, giving the sibling (or father) listed on the calendar a day's reprieve.

When we began this practice, Niel was still a little too short to reach into the sink, so he had to stand on a short stool to do the dishes. If it was Ken's turn, he had to leave his leg braces on until after dinner, and stand, balancing on his crutches and braces to do the work. In retrospect, I am amazed that he continued to do this faithfully for several years without complaining because this was fairly difficult for him. However, he believed that he needed to do his share of dishwashing to be fair and to be a good example.

It was a good thing that Ken managed this chore the way he did because the dishwashing schedule became a very big deal for our kids. They were always checking with the calendar to see who was named for duty that day, chortling with glee when it was not their turn and teasing the unlucky sibling who did have that responsibility. There was also quite a bit of protesting and teasing when one of them slipped up and had more than three rejects, giving a sibling or their dad a free pass for the next evening.

Probably the most impressive duty that Ken took on with our children was doing the grocery shopping every three to four weeks; he started this when they were about twelve, eleven, and nine. For the first few trips, I accompanied the family so they could learn which brands and sizes I usually purchased. When Ken and our children went out to shop, he divided the grocery list, giving part of it to Diane, who took a cart of her own and gathered the items on her list. Ken walked around the store on his crutches and braces, with one of the boys pushing a cart and both of them picking up the items as he called them out and then marked them off his list. With a little practice, this system worked surprisingly well, and it did save me a great deal of time.

Ken's mom and dad were also a very important source of help during this period, especially when I took two or more classes at a time or needed classes that were only available during the day. In the fall of 1969, Elsie and Emil moved out of Chicago and into an apartment in St. Charles. Emil was concerned about his continuing ability to drive and about Elsie's well-being. She had had a serious stroke earlier that year and had not regained some of her ability to function. Obviously, if they lived closer to us, we would be better able to help them when they needed it.

Truth be told, for the first several years after they moved, I think they helped us quite a bit more than we helped them. As I started taking more courses and had to be away from home for longer periods of time, they filled in the gaps, making sure that Diane, Brian, and Niel had adult supervision and were able to get home safely from school. It was a win-win situation. They and our children enjoyed having more time together, and Ken and I were relieved to know that they had reliable backup supervision.

The year they moved, Ken received some good and unexpected news at Argonne. With just a little additional coursework, which he could complete at Argonne with pay, he could finish the requirements for the doctoral degree he had chosen to set aside in 1961 when he learned that I was pregnant. Argonne National Laboratory was (and still is) administered by the University of Chicago, working for the Department of Energy, and one of the administrative objectives at the time was to increase the number of researchers employed at Argonne who had doctoral degrees. Ken lacked just two or three courses and had not formally written or defended a doctoral dissertation. However, he had already published substantial articles based upon his own original research that were equivalent to a dissertation in their content. All he had to do was to complete the coursework and "defend" one of the research articles he was currently finishing before a doctoral committee! He finished these requirements in July of 1970, thereby earning a PhD in Applied Mathematics from the University of Chicago.

Even though this was a significant achievement, Ken chose to interpret it primarily as yet another indication of the Lord's amazing faithfulness, not that he had accomplished anything that remarkable. He was thankful for the promotion and increase in salary that accompanied it but chiefly because that helped him better provide for his family. I think he also told Elsie the news, but I don't remember him telling anyone else. In fact, when he learned that he would have to pay fifty dollars to have his diploma printed so it could be nicely displayed, he decided that the money would be better spent on family needs and chose not to order it. I didn't know that he had made that decision until much later.

Contrary to what it might appear, our life together during the years I was working toward the BA was not all toil and seriousness. During a lot of that time, I took courses at a slow pace and made it a priority to keep my summers free from study. I also gave my family a break and resumed most of the housework myself during the summer months. We had made a number of friends at our church, and Ken and I met regularly with a small group known as the "Homebuilders," couples about our age who still had children at home. We also enjoyed occasional potluck dinners and picnics with other church members and their families.

By this time, there were several other families living in our subdivision, so our children had other children they went to school with and played with at home. A few years after we moved, we set up a swing set with a slide and a glider, and they and their friends spent many hours enjoying that equipment. In nice weather, it was difficult to get them to come inside at a reasonable hour to take their baths and get ready for bed.

Sometimes they wandered off our property and onto nearby vacant lots. On the back of the lot just north of us, there was a sizable thicket of blackberry bushes (which have sharp thorns) that particularly fascinated our kids. For reasons I was never fully able to appreciate, Diane and Brian decided that this would be a perfect place to build a "fort." They had watched me use my pruners to cut back shrubs and reasoned that they could borrow these to hollow out a narrow entrance and hidden inner rooms in this tangle of briars. They made the "floor" more tolerable by lining it with a thick layer of grass clippings.

By the time it was finished, they had, indeed, constructed a formidable fort! No adult, or faint-hearted child, for that matter, would dare to enter it! However, when all three children started coming in from play with some serious scratches and bleeding pinpricks on their arms and legs, I noticed and they had to "fess up" to their covert activities. Secretly, I had to admire their ingenuity and persistence. However, I had to discourage further fort development in the blackberry thicket because of the injuries it was inflicting. After quite a few additional pinpricks and scratches, they eventually came to the same conclusion.

In the winter, our three would go outside in the snow and build forts, make snowmen, dig tunnels in tall drifts, sled or ski down the hill in our backyard, and engage in family or group snowball fights with other children. I always provided them with boots, mittens, and snowsuits to make sure they would stay warm. On one of their very early forays out into the snow, when Niel was about two, I bundled them up in their gear and told them to play close to the house. However, they were not outside very long until Diane and Brian came running in, very excited and upset, to tell me that Niel was stuck in a snowdrift! Since I couldn't walk very well through deep snow myself, I had to shovel out a fairly long path for myself to rescue him. He had apparently walked on top of a fresh drift that collapsed under his weight, and he had fallen in, right up to his armpits. In his bulky snowsuit, he simply couldn't climb out by himself! He was upset by his predicament but not hurt. When I shared the incident with Ken that evening, we all had a good laugh, and Niel's misadventure became one of our family classics.

When Brian and Niel were old enough, they played Little League baseball in the summer. In between these games, they sometimes organized informal ball games with friends or simply practiced batting and catching in the open areas of the yard. Sometimes Ken, Diane, and I would join them. Amazingly, Ken discovered a way to swing the bat effectively with just his right arm while seated in his wheelchair. One of our children would pitch the ball to him or he would toss it into the air himself and send it flying with considerable height and distance, providing good catching practice for those stationed in the outfield. My batting and throwing performances were pretty pathetic because of lingering weakness in my right triceps muscles from polio, so I usually stood on the sidelines, cheering the others on or retrieving stray balls for Ken.

Our family life in those earlier years was also enlivened by a series of noteworthy pets. Early on, Ken wanted a dog, so we purchased a very friendly Golden Retriever puppy. We named him Samson, anticipating that he would become a powerful specimen in maturity. He certainly lived up to those expectations! He enjoyed taking me for brisk (and risky) walks every time I had him on a leash. In the winter, he loved to join our children in their play and to plow through fresh snowdrifts at top speed, sending the snow flying in all directions.

At another time, we purchased two brash little parakeets we named Pete and Repeat because they looked so much alike we could never tell them apart. They loved to sound off at high volume whenever anyone tried to talk on the telephone that was located just across from them in the family room. This was also where we ate our meals, and they would sometimes chime in on our dinner conversations as well. We had several goldfish, but they all seemed to have a death wish. We would have them for a while, but they would invariably jump out of the tank and onto the carpet to an untimely death. There were also assorted cats and kittens that we brought home with us from the farm after summer visits with my family. One infamous pair we named Bonny and Clyde, because of the number of mice they killed and then brought into the garage, leaving many of these as trophies for us to see (and obstacles for us to remove) on the ramp leading into the house.

Ken was fortunate to have a generous number of vacation days from his work each year, so we also took frequent trips together during the summer. Some of these were shorter sight-seeing trips into Missouri, Wisconsin, along Lake Michigan or Lake Superior, or into Chicago. Many of our trips were downstate visits to my parents and extended family. These were enjoyable for Ken because of his enduring fascination with farms and farming and with varied scenery and people to visit and photograph. I was always grateful to be able to spend time with my family. Our children were eager to visit because they were about the same ages as my youngest brothers and sister and they always found new and exciting things to do when they were all together.

On these trips, we would also set aside time to visit with my grandmother and two of her sisters who also lived in the area. Visiting my grandmother and my step-grandfather at their house in Barry would always bring back fond memories of the years I had lived there as a child, of Grandmother's unfailing love and concern for me and my sister and her admonitions that we needed to believe in Jesus. We would also visit Aunt Naomi and Uncle Claude, who had helped me a little financially and encouraged me a great deal during my first two years at the U of I. It was always somewhat humorous to see the two of them standing side by side because of the great disparity in their heights. Aunt Naomi could stand erect, quite comfortably, right under my uncle's outstretched arm!

One of the places that our children really enjoyed visiting was Aunt Wilma and Uncle Russell's farm, located a couple of miles from my parents' property. The prim white farmhouse, red barns, and sheds were all nestled in a beautiful little valley surrounded by rolling hills on all sides. In front of the house, about fifteen yards from the front gate, was a meandering, spring-fed creek, and right behind the creek was a steep densely wooded hillside punctuated at intervals with weathered outcroppings of rock. Former residents had built a picturesque "spring house" into the hillside, right over part of the creek, taking advantage of the ice-cold spring water to create a natural refrigerator for milk and other foods.

Aunt Wilma had surrounded their farmhouse with flowers and gardens and transformed the wide front porch into a magical place to sit and talk. She had planted a honeysuckle vine at one end of the porch, which grew right up to the roof, and had Uncle Russell install a porch swing in front of it. Two or three people could sit in the swing, relax, converse, listen to the rustling water in the creek, smell the honeysuckle, and watch the hummingbirds that frequently visited the flowers during their long season of bloom.

The feature that really fascinated our children on these visits, besides a creek to play in, was Uncle Russell's riding horses. He enjoyed riding and showing his horses at local fairs and horse shows and had saddles and other gear for each one. He would frequently invite guests to ride along with him and enjoy the scenic beauty of his property. He also loved children, and when our children came to visit, they were always offered an opportunity to ride the horses. Diane and Brian both had opportunity for more extended summer visits to the farm when they were a little older. Among other unusual activities, they learned how to safely gather eggs from under cranky, possessive hens, how to handle and shoot a rifle, and how to skin and dress squirrels for human consumption.

The year I was finishing my bachelor's degree, Ken and I both started praying for guidance about what I should do after it was completed. One option was to seek employment right away. However, doing so would probably mean that I would not be doing work related to my major. Counseling, teaching, or working in industry in the field of psychology required a masters or doctoral degree. The other option was to begin graduate work at NIU. I had done exceptionally well in my undergraduate courses, and as we sought guidance, we both had a strong sense that I should continue with graduate training, right to a PhD. As he had been all along, Ken was strongly supportive and keen to help me achieve this goal. I planned to seek part-time work as a graduate assistant to reduce the cost of my education and to start taking courses at a much faster pace. My goal was to be finished and employed by the time our children were ready for college.

Proceeding on in graduate work was actually not that different from what I had been doing my last semester as a full-time undergraduate. We already had a system of family cooperation in place that gave me adequate time to study. Emil and Elsie were quite willing to continue to help. In addition, full-time graduate study actually gave me more flexibility and time at home than if I had started a full-time job. Not only that, I realized that by managing my time carefully, we could still use part of our summers to travel and to do things together as a family.

I received my bachelor's degree in January of 1972 and used the spring semester to take a couple of graduate courses and to plan the research I needed for a master's thesis. The idea for this research actually came from hearing of Elsie's experiences with hyperthyroidism. When Ken was about ten, Elsie's thyroid gland enlarged and began secreting larger and larger amounts of thyroid hormone. In addition to physical symptoms, such as increasing body temperature and weight loss, she also began to experience disruptive anxiety attacks and irrational phobias. Shortly after her physical condition was corrected by surgery, the anxieties and phobias also diminished greatly without psychological intervention.

There were similar case studies in the medical literature, and I wondered if this effect could be replicated experimentally in laboratory rats. There was already a well-established experimental procedure for measuring fear behavior in rats, and the professor I was working for at the time also had the necessary equipment. However, before I could test my hypothesis, I needed to establish a physiologically effective dose of thyroxin for the rats. This required a pilot study that I received permission to carry out at home—systematically administering different doses of thyroxin and watching for small but reliable increases in the rat's basal metabolic rates.

This pilot study wasn't difficult, but it meant keeping twenty white rats in cages in our utility room for several weeks. While I was in the midst of this study, our kids were very intrigued and curious, but what they seemed to enjoy the most was telling all of their neighborhood friends about all the rats we had in the house! Perhaps incidents like this help explain why psychologists are sometimes considered a bit strange. (Incidentally, in the actual research and in a follow-up study, I did find that rats with increased thyroxin levels behaved like they were more fearful than control rats that received a similar placebo.)

An important decision I had to make early in my graduate training was choosing the area of psychology in which to specialize. As I considered what the Lord might want me to do, I first thought of clinical psychology or counseling since these involved helping other people. This area also offered the most opportunities for employment. However, after taking a couple of clinical courses at NIU, I knew this wasn't the right direction. I tried, but I could not get excited about what I was learning, partly because the therapies and techniques were based on completely secular models of human nature and partly because I just wasn't interested in learning to apply various therapeutic techniques.

I was most enthusiastic when studying the incredibly intricate way our bodies and brains had been created, the way they functioned, the mystery of human consciousness and self-awareness, and the way physical events in the brain and body appeared to be related to our conscious experiences. These were exciting to me because each new discovery or insight revealed more about God, His intricate care in creating us, His infinite wisdom and capability, and His obvious love and provision for us. Learning about the possible causes of anxiety disorders, depression, schizophrenia, and the effects of brain damage was also fascinating.

At this point, it was not clear what the Lord had in mind for me to do with the particular skills and interests He had given me.

Whatever it was, I was determined to choose a specialization that would allow me to find employment and to find it reasonably close to home. Ken had a well-established career at Argonne, our children loved their home and friends, and I certainly didn't want to uproot any of that for the sake of my career. Looking back, I can see that my excessive concern about finding a job (as opposed to trusting that the Lord was already working out those arrangements) effectively blinded me to other career possibilities like teaching, in which job opportunities were much more limited. I finally decided that something at least related to clinical psychology—perhaps doing research into the causes of psychopathology—was what I should pursue.

My academic advisor thought this idea was reasonable and suggested that I take a broad, wide-ranging mix of academic psychology courses including neuroscience, cognition, research methods, etc. and selected courses in psychopathology. He also encouraged me to do an internship with schizophrenic patients, under his supervision, at a local facility. This lineup of courses didn't match any of the specializations in psychology that were offered at NIU, but I could get around that by specializing in my advisor's area of training, personality/social psychology, which had a small number of required courses. If I took the required courses and passed the comprehensive exams in that area, he would give me the latitude to take whatever other courses I felt I needed. I discussed this with Ken, accepted his offer, and then set to work on my studies in earnest, encouraged that I was still heading in the right direction.

Chapter 10

God's Provision

With the Lord's help and the continuing support of my family, I was able to progress through graduate study at NIU at an efficient pace. By January of 1974, I had finished the master's degree, and by the fall of 1975, I had completed my coursework, was working part-time in the dean's office, and was conducting research for the dissertation. It was also time to begin a job search. That prospect created some anxiety because, at that time, career opportunities outside the fields of clinical or counseling psychology were very limited. Some of the other PhD candidates I knew who were not in clinical specializations were actually sending out resumes across the entire United States and even beyond. I was limiting my search to within forty miles of home! I tried not to think about the apparent odds against me and to leave the matter in God's hands, but I still felt some anxiety.

A few weeks into that semester, I received word from my advisor, Dr. Martin, that Wheaton College would be seeking doctoral candidates for the position of Assistant Professor for the next academic year. He was aware of this only because the professor who was vacating that position at Wheaton had mentioned it in passing to one of his former professors at NIU, who then shared it with other faculty. Dr. Martin knew that Wheaton required their faculty to be Christians, and he was aware of my beliefs, so he encouraged me to apply.

This news immediately captured my attention. I thought about Ken's long and meaningful connection with Wheaton College and how we had visited the campus on several occasions, wondering if someday we might be able to send our own children there. Wheaton was also only twenty-five miles from our home— a reasonable commute. Could this be the Lord's guidance? At first, I was hesitant because I simply hadn't considered teaching as a profession. The possibility of finding such a position within my search area had seemed much too remote. For some reason, which I couldn't even remember, I had also vowed earlier in my life never to become a teacher. However, I had enjoyed occasionally teaching Sunday school classes at church and instructing undergraduates as a teaching assistant. As I considered this possibility, it rapidly became more appealing.

When Ken came home from work that afternoon, I shared the news with him, and he too immediately sensed that we might be seeing God's hand in this. The next day, I called the college and indicated my interest in applying for the position. The personnel office sent me the necessary paperwork, and after two or three weeks they gave me a call and invited me to schedule an interview.

The interviewing process was very thorough, stretching over two full days and requiring me to talk with many people, including the president of the college, the Faculty Personnel Committee, the chairman and other members of the Psychology Department, plus a group of psychology majors. I was also asked to teach a seminar on my own research or a topic of interest that would then be evaluated by some of the faculty and students. These interactions gave me opportunity to ask my own questions and to meet potential colleagues.

I was not that aware of it when I interviewed, but I did differ in some significant ways from the majority of professors employed at Wheaton. For one, I had a fairly minor but occasionally obvious physical disability. I could walk and stand fairly normally, but I needed to carry and utilize a cane-like crutch to step up curbs or to climb flights of stairs. Secondly, the overwhelming majority of the faculty were men. Among women faculty, there was only one or two who were married and had children living at home. (When I interviewed, there was a legitimate concern that the heavy teaching load might force a woman who also had the primary responsibility of taking care of children and a home to neglect either her family or her job.) I was also different in that I had not grown up in the church. I hadn't even become a Christian until I was twenty-three. Some of these issues surfaced from time to time during my interviews, but they didn't seem important at the time.

Two interviews remain especially vivid. One was meeting with the department chair and discovering that the unconventional set of graduate courses that I had taken and even the research I had engaged in had prepared me very well to teach the undergraduate courses that were needed, even down to minor details like helping students work with laboratory rats. Most significantly, I would also be responsible for developing and teaching a new interdisciplinary course in neuroscience, the study of the interrelationships between physiological events in our bodies and brains and our conscious capabilities and experiences. This area of study was my absolute favorite!

The other unforgettable interview was meeting with President Hudson T. Armerding. He was a tall, lean man with a dignified bearing that he had evidently acquired from his military training and service as an officer in the United States Navy during and after World War II. He welcomed me into his office, and I immediately sensed that he was a very capable and godly man. I instantly liked and respected him. He was very kind and gracious, but he also came right to the point with his questions. One that he asked early in the interview was how I would manage a heavy teaching schedule with three teenagers still at home. I thought that was a legitimate question and was certainly not put off by it. I told him that I would do it with the Lord's help and with the same cooperation from my family that had enabled me to get through graduate school. I explained that our children had learned to help and to take responsibility at home while they were quite young and that they also understood that an important reason I was working was to help them get a college education. This struck a responsive chord, and I could tell that Dr. Armerding was surprised but also pleased with this explanation.

As I drove home after that second day, I reviewed the remarkable chain of events that were linking up—my "accidental" discovery that a position at Wheaton was available right when I was prepared to apply for it, Ken's past connections with Wheaton, the match between my training and interests and what I would be teaching, and even the reasonable commute. It seemed that my interviews and the seminar had gone reasonable well. As I reflected on these things, I had the very strong impression that I was witnessing God's remarkable and tangible guidance. So by the time I pulled into our driveway that afternoon, I was fairly confident that I would get the position—not so much because of my qualifications but rather because of my assurance that the Lord was guiding this process. I knew it would be some time before I heard from Wheaton because they were also interviewing other candidates for the position. In the meantime, I turned my attention back to my family's needs and working on the dissertation.

The weeks went by, and we celebrated Thanksgiving together, but there was still no word from Wheaton College. Ken, Elsie, and I kept praying about the situation, and they both remained confident that the position at Wheaton was what God had prepared me for. However, I was getting concerned. That concern grew stronger when three more weeks passed by with no word. Finally, right before Christmas, I received a letter. However, as I scanned it, I could hardly believe what I was reading! Wheaton had offered the position to two other candidates "who seemed best able to meet our current needs." And although neither candidate had accepted the position yet, they wanted to advise me of their actions without any further delay.

That news was very upsetting for several reasons. For one, I immediately interpreted the letter to mean that the opportunity at Wheaton was gone, because I couldn't imagine that both candidates would turn down this position in a very tight job market. I was also confused because I had sensed the Lord's leading so strongly. Had I totally misinterpreted my situation and manufactured that sense of assurance myself? Even worse, had my premature enthusiasm also misled Ken and Elsie? Could I even trust such feelings again?

In marked contrast to my bewilderment, Ken and Elsie remained upbeat. They simply didn't believe that this was the way the future would unfold! They were veterans of some very tough spiritual battles and had faced numerous "impossible" obstacles together during Ken's long recovery from polio and his intense struggle to get an education. Their reasons for not conceding to what I thought was inevitable were simple—God doesn't deal arbitrarily with His children!

I was very grateful for their encouragement and continuing support during that period because the news precipitated a deep spiritual crisis in me that took some weeks to resolve. While interviewing, it had seemed obvious that the Holy Spirit was giving me strong assurances of guidance and exciting reasons for all those years of study. However, the letter seemed to indicate that I had been mistaken. More questions followed. Did I truly have a genuine relationship with the Lord? And even, at my lowest point, was He just a creation of my mind? Had I essentially just been yielding to my old, selfish ambition and making the effort seem good to others by framing it as the Lord's will?

Christmas that year was subdued, even though I tried hard to make it festive. I couldn't reconcile the conflicting information in my mind. I didn't linger on those doubts about God because I knew that He was real, that He loved me, and that He had guided both Ken and me in many remarkable ways. However, I still had serious questions about the legitimacy of my fourteen-year quest for a PhD. I wrapped presents, prepared an elegant Christmas dinner, and did everything I could to make the day a celebration, but my family knew I was struggling.

Spring semester commenced, and I realized that I had to get in gear and finish my dissertation, even if I didn't know what the future might bring. One morning before my first appointment in the dean's office, I started fretting again. I quickly pulled a Bible out of my desk drawer, thinking that reading it would help me regain some focus. However, instead of going to a specific passage, I just thumbed halfheartedly through pages and for no particular reason stopped near the end of 1 Peter, in chapter 5. I started reading at verse 5, *"God opposes the proud but gives grace to the humble."* This caught my attention and I read on:

> *Humble yourselves, therefore, under God's mighty hand, that he may lift you up in due time. Cast all your anxiety on him because he cares for you. Be self-controlled and alert. Your enemy the devil prowls around like a roaring lion looking for someone to devour. Resist him, standing firm in the faith, because you know that your brothers throughout the world are undergoing the same kind of sufferings.*
>
> *And the God of all grace, who called you to his eternal glory in Christ, after you have suffered a little while, will himself restore you and make you strong, firm and steadfast. To him be the power for ever and ever. Amen.*

As I was puzzling over this passage, wondering if it might apply to my situation, a vivid but seemingly unrelated question formed in my mind. "Betty, do you still trust Me?" I was startled by its clarity and directness but could honestly answer, "Yes, I still trust

You." Then another question, "Would you still trust Me even if you didn't get the position at Wheaton College?" This question was puzzling because I had already concluded that this issue was settled, so I didn't have to think about it long. "Yes, Lord. I trust You even though I do not understand what happened in that situation." Then a third question, "Would you still trust me if you could *never* find employment commensurate with your education?" This question alarmed me and was difficult for me to affirm. If that were to happen, how would I ever explain it—to myself, my family, or others who had prayed with me and helped me during all those years of study. I really didn't want events to turn out that way and didn't want to somehow "give God permission" to let such a thing happen. After some moments of turmoil, I started reviewing what I knew about God from the Bible: God is sovereign, God is good, and in all things He works for the good of those who love Him, who are called according to His purpose. With these assurances in mind, I was able to answer "Yes, I will still trust You."

I looked back at the Scripture I had been reading and lingered on the phrase, *"God opposes the proud."* It was then that I realized that I had actually become proud of my academic achievements and had even started thinking that God was affirming my ability and diligence in study by rewarding me with a teaching position at Wheaton College—that I somehow deserved that position. Because of my inflated pride, learning that I was in third place or lower among the candidates who interviewed was a painful but beneficial blow. My attitude had been very wrong. If God calls us to a position of responsibility, we are to consider it a privilege and an opportunity to serve, in obedience to God and for the sake of those we are serving, not as an opportunity to build up status or impress other people. I needed to repent and destroy this ugly idol. In reality, I would not have been able to accomplish any of what I had done without all of the loving patience and assistance from my family and God's consistent help and guidance.

These insights and my heart-felt repentance brought a strong and lasting sense of peace, and I was finally able to shift my attention totally to the tasks at hand. I didn't even sense a need to begin my search for employment right away. Several weeks later, while I was doing some mending at my sewing machine, the telephone rang, and I was very surprised when the caller identified himself as the Vice President for Academic Affairs at Wheaton College. He was calling me about the position for Assistant Professor. He was very apologetic about calling after I had been sent a letter of rejection, but he explained that a number of "very unusual" circumstances had taken place and that both of the candidates who had been offered the position had turned it down. Through all this, he and others overseeing the selection process had concluded that the Lord was trying to tell them something. He then asked me if I would be willing to reconsider taking the position myself!

I was so surprised and had such difficulty trying to assimilate what he was saying that I was simply at a loss for words. In the smallness of my faith, I had concluded that this opportunity was gone, and now I could scarcely believe that it was back. I finally managed to stammer that I needed to think and pray about this decision and that I would call him back. Ken was at home, and when I shared this news with him, he was pleased but not as surprised by this turn of events as he was at my response to the vice president. He told me, "Betty, what are you waiting for? This is obviously the Lord's provision that we have all been praying for. Get back on that phone and accept the offer!" I did, and as they say, the rest is history.

I signed a contract in March of 1976 to start teaching full-time in September of 1976. When I signed, I agreed that I would try to finish my dissertation before the fall semester started. In the five intervening months, I also needed to organize and set up the five classes I was to teach that school year, create schedules, choose and order textbooks, and start preparing lectures. And as if that were not enough, shortly after signing, I was also informed by our family physician that I needed a complete hysterectomy as soon as I could manage it. I had been under medical treatment for severe endometriosis for more than a year, but that treatment hadn't worked. Since laparoscopic techniques were not yet available, I was also facing an extended recovery period.

I could have felt overwhelmed, but at that point, I knew without a doubt that it was the Lord who had opened the door for me to teach at Wheaton. That being the case, I could also count on Him to give me the healing and extra strength and endurance I would need to meet all of my commitments on time. Thankfully, I also knew that I had Ken's and our family's unwavering support. Since I wouldn't be able to drive for a while after the surgery, I needed to complete the work that had to be done at NIU (data analysis, additional library research, etc.) before the operation. I could then have the surgery in late May and write the dissertation and work on my new courses at home while I was recovering.

This strategy worked, but at several points I ran frighteningly short of time. For instance, I was able to finish writing the dissertation and take the last pages to the typist just the day before I needed to be at Wheaton College for new-faculty orientation and last-minute preparations for classes! In addition, I successfully defended the dissertation later that fall in the midst of my first semester of teaching and was granted the PhD in December. That year, 1976, had been one of the most demanding and difficult years of my life, but it was also a time of incredible spiritual growth and strengthening as I watched the Lord help me meet one tough challenge after another.

Teaching at Wheaton was at once exciting, fulfilling, and demanding. Even in that hectic first year, I enjoyed teaching, preparing for classes, and working with highly motivated students and colleagues who shared the same worldview and served the same Lord. The change in atmosphere from that of NIU was especially stark. During all my years as a graduate student there, I did not meet another classmate or professor who gave clear evidence of being a Christ follower. I could also see that teaching effectively would be a challenge and wasn't likely to grow stale. There would probably always be room for innovation and improvement!

My transition from student to teacher was exciting for me and good for our family. Preparing for classes, teaching, grading, keeping office hours, and meeting other responsibilities consumed more than forty hours a week on most weeks, but my schedule was also more flexible. I needed to be on campus only three or four days a week and could do a lot of my preparation at home. Since teaching during the summer was not a requirement, I used some of that time to update lectures, enrich classes, and catch up on new developments in my field. The extra flexibility also allowed me to take over much of the housework and maintain a consistent schedule of family meals. Another benefit, which Ken really appreciated, was the possibility of extended travel. We now had the time plus an extra income to work with.

By this time Diane, Brian, and Niel were fifteen, fourteen, and twelve and were themselves interested in longer, scenic trips. However the costs of staying in motels and eating at restaurants would add up quickly. Camping was appealing because we had seen some beautiful campgrounds on previous trips and knew that traveling this way could be more economical and enjoyable. Tent camping obviously wouldn't work, but camping with a trailer might be possible if it could be made accessible and had suitable bathroom, kitchen, and sleeping facilities. With these, we could stay in scenic campgrounds in state and national parks overnight and prepare our own food. And if we wanted to explore, we could simply unhitch and leave the trailer in the campsite.

Traveling with a trailer would pose some difficulties. I would be preparing most of our meals, but this wasn't a big issue because I knew these could be simple. There was also the problem of hitching, unhitching, and leveling the trailer. Neither Ken nor I could do this, but Brian and Niel were both strong, mechanically adept, and willing, so we were reasonably sure they could handle the job. A more serious concern was the feasibility of safely maneuvering and towing a good-sized trailer across the country while driving with hand controls, sometimes in less-than-optimal conditions. However, by this time, both of us had many years of experience driving this way and were fairly confident that we could manage safely.

We went shopping and found a trailer that met most of our needs. It was twenty-five-feet long and had three compartments, one with a double bed and a small bathroom, a second furnished with four bunk beds, and a third with a kitchen and dining area. There was a problem with the entrance, which was fairly high and which was accessed by one, narrow, retractable step. Using this step to get into the trailer was difficult for me and impossible for Ken. He could not manage this with his crutches and braces. We solved this problem by constructing a portable, light-weight set of wooden steps that our teens could set in place as needed.

Shortly after purchasing the trailer, we took a five-day trip to Barry to visit, obtain driving practice, and to check out all the systems and appliances. Driving was slower and required more concentration with the trailer in tow, so it was also more tiring, especially when there was rain or moderate wind to contend with. We discovered that we needed to think about how we would exit each potential stopping place before pulling into it with the trailer since backing out was difficult. We also learned to stop at larger stations when we needed gas or to fill up while the trailer was unhitched. Trying to get safely in and out of smaller gas stations with the trailer could be problematic.

We made that first trip safely, managing to pull the trailer up the long, steep, gravel road leading to my parents' farm, and then backing it into a level spot near the farmhouse. However, our first night together in the trailer was anything but routine. Ken and I slept in the back compartment, Diane and Brian slept in the two lower bunk beds in the next compartment, and Niel slept in the bunk right above Brian's. The beds were comfortable and we were tired, so we all fell asleep fairly quickly that night. Somewhere around midnight, Ken and I were rudely awakened by a lot of loud, angry yelling coming from the middle compartment. I struggled to get out of bed in darkness and unfamiliar surroundings to find out what was going on. Niel had evidently had a bad dream, started yelling loudly in his sleep, and jumped out of his upper bunk, landing partly on top of Diane in her bunk across the aisle. Diane was startled out of a sound sleep and angered by her brother's painful intrusion, and she started yelling too. In the meantime, Brian woke up and started scolding his sibs, upset that he had been awakened by their uproar.

Strangely, in the midst of all this mayhem, Niel did not wake up. Shortly after Diane started protesting, he scrambled out of her bunk without a word and climbed right back up into his bunk and stretched out, sound asleep. While the rest of us were marveling at Niel's apparent obliviousness, I heard a soft knock on the trailer door and opened it to see Mom standing outside in her robe. She looked pretty worried and asked me softly, "Is everything all right?" Her bedroom was not far from the trailer, and she was sleeping with her window open, so all of the commotion had jolted her awake. I can't imagine what she thought might be going on, but I quickly explained what had happened and then we all started laughing—except for Niel, who was still sound asleep! He had no recollection of the episode the next morning!

The successful trip downstate and more experience with the trailer that summer gave us the confidence we needed to plan a much longer trip for the next year. Finally, in 1978, ten years after our first attempt at a long family vacation, we were headed back to the west and the Rocky Mountains. This time all of us were eager to travel and see new places. Ken drew upon his extensive knowledge of scenic places and national parks and planned a stunning, twenty-eight-day trip that took us to many remarkable areas, including, among others, Rocky Mountain National Park, the Trail Ridge Road, the Grand Tetons, Jenny Lake, and Yellowstone.

This time we drove fewer miles each day and were able to enjoy the journey as well as the destinations, staying at some interesting campgrounds on the way. We used extra time at campsites to explore, talk with other campers, or to play cards or board games as a family. Moreover, because we had our own familiar "bed and breakfast" with us, we didn't have to be concerned about accessibility in motel rooms or with finding suitable places to eat each night.

Not too surprisingly, since we were still novices with the trailer, we did run into a few unexpected glitches on this trip—two of them fairly serious. In the first situation, we pulled into an attractive state park campground and discovered that the only camping spaces that were long enough for our station wagon and trailer were curved "pullouts." These were short paved areas that curved off the main road, straightened out for a distance, and then curved back onto the main road again. Ken was driving, and we spotted one pullout that was long and nicely shaded. What neither of us thought about until we were well into that space was that the first curve went right between two large trees, one a few feet in front of the other. By the time we realized that this space was too tight for the trailer, we were in a bind. It didn't look like we could pull out or back out without scraping against one of the trees.

I couldn't see a solution, and Diane and I nearly panicked. However, Ken and Brian and Niel, evidently better equipped to visualize a solution than we were, started working on the problem together. Both boys got out, Brian on one side of the trailer and Niel on the other, so they could help Ken inch the trailer back and forth without scraping the trees until he finally maneuvered into a position that allowed him to get out. This took a long time (at least it seemed that way to me), so we all felt a lot of relief and a bit frazzled by the time we could pull away. This taught us to drive around and scrutinize available campsites very carefully before we tried to park.

The other, potentially more serious incident occurred close to Yellowstone Park while I was driving. We were once again following directions to get to a campground, and I turned off the paved road onto a gravel road that would take us to our destination. I noticed that the gravel on this road was loose, and we both saw that we were going to have to pull the trailer up a long, steep hill. Ken suggested that I shift into second gear and keep the speed fairly slow but steady because we could already feel our back wheels spinning a little in the loose gravel. I made it to the top of the hill, but just as the hill leveled off, the road made an abrupt T-intersection with a second road. Since it wasn't immediately apparent whether I should go right or left, I made the mistake of pausing, ever so briefly. When I did accelerate a little to make the turn, the back wheels started spinning and throwing the loose gravel. I tried several times to move forward, to no avail. We were stuck! The only thing we could do was to try to back down this steep slope as carefully as possible. There were significant drop offs on both sides of the road, but fortunately the road was fairly wide, so there was some room for error. Both of us were praying silently but fervently that the Lord would help us get out of this predicament safely.

Ken was far better at backing the trailer than I, so I set the brakes and we carefully switched places. Diane, Brian, and Niel got out and stood along both sides of the road so they could signal Ken via the side mirrors or by voice if he was getting too close to the edge of the road. Once again, I really had to admire Ken's courage under pressure. Putting the station wagon in reverse, using the hand controls and the mirrors, with one hand on the brake and the other on the steering wheel, he slowly and skillfully guided the trailer back down that long hill to safety. After that incident, we caught our breath and then headed to a different campground!

Even though these two incidents gave us pause, they did not diminish our overall enjoyment of this trip and the time we spent together. It was very satisfying to park in beautiful settings, to eat together in the comfort of our own dwelling, and to prepare for the night at a leisurely pace. It was enjoyable to experience dusk and the different night sounds in new places and to stare up at the myriad blazing stars in remote locations. For Ken, it was especially meaningful to be able to actually stay in places he had always longed to experience more intimately. It was also gratifying for him to be able to share his fascination with the beauty and wonder of God's creation with our nearly grown children and to see their own increasing appreciation of these things as well.

Experiences like these made Ken think back to the promise that he had received from God while he was struggling for his life and his faith in that iron lung so many years before. "You will live, and your life will be very meaningful." With the overwhelming physical limitations that he had at that time, how could he have possibly imagined that one day he would have an excellent education, a meaningful career, a wife and family, and a home, and that he would also be able to travel, actually camping with his family in remote and beautiful areas that he had often longed to visit. He could only conclude that God had indeed provided for him in amazing ways and had been completely faithful to His promises.

Chapter 11

Challenges and Changes

F inishing school and finding employment at Wheaton College ended one very significant chapter in our lives and marked the beginning of another, filled with its own unique blessings and struggles. The next fourteen years was a time of fulfillment and stability for Ken and me but a time of significant change for our family. During that time, our children became adults, left home, married, and started families of their own. And as Elsie and Emil grew older and less able, they became increasingly dependent upon us for help. Their need became acute during my first year of teaching.

Emil had always been somewhat difficult to get along with, but as he aged, he also became bitter and more openly prejudiced. Shortly before I began teaching, the manager at Emil's apartment complex asked him to move out as soon as his lease expired. He had made offensive remarks to some of the minority maintenance workers and tenants there. Apparently word of his poor behavior also spread to other apartment owners—no one I called was willing to rent to Emil. This created a serious problem. We didn't have room to bring both Elsie and Emil into our home, long term, and we were sure that Emil's presence would be extremely and consistently disruptive.

This situation was particularly difficult for Ken. At first he was absolutely furious that Emil's poor behavior had once again put him in a very difficult situation. Ken had never truly forgiven Emil for his excessive drinking, his poor treatment of Elsie, or his earlier abandonment. After Emil had moved out, Ken had stopped calling him "Dad" and from that point forward would only address him as "Emil." Ken's inner struggle with his anger and frustration was so deep that he didn't want to discuss it or pray about it with me. He knew he was reacting poorly but also believed that this was something he had to settle, one on one, between himself and the Lord. After a few days, Ken grew calmer and told me that the Lord had definitely shown him what we should do. Unless I had strong objections against it, we needed to step out in faith and purchase a second, smaller house so his parents would have a place to live!

Ken was still disturbed by the situation but was determined to obey because the Lord's answer had come through as a "command." By his own description, it was as clear as the words of encouragement the Lord had given him when he was struggling with polio and as his conviction, on our first meeting, that I was the person he would marry. This situation with Emil was the third time that the Lord had communicated with him so clearly and directly.

In retrospect, I believe there were at least three objectives the Lord had in mind for this instruction besides insuring that Emil and Elsie would have a suitable place to live. One was to help Ken come to terms with his anger and lack of forgiveness. A second was helping all of us grow in compassion, patience, and a willingness to serve others. A third was to teach Ken and me to trust God more fully for our financial security. Initially Ken was reluctant to purchase a second house because he didn't think it was fair to me or our children. If we took this step, we would be signing for a second mortgage while still paying off our first! Moreover, our teenagers were rapidly approaching college age with all the expenses that would entail.

As long as his fears and worries had the upper hand, all Ken could think about was how could we possibly pay all of those bills. However, after he accepted the fact that purchasing a second house was the Lord's will and started working with the numbers, he realized that there were factors he had overlooked that would greatly reduce our risk. For one, Elsie and Emil could apply the money they had been paying for rent to the monthly mortgage payments. For another, we now had two incomes to work with, and for yet a third, we were in good shape with our own mortgage and credit because Ken had been steadily prepaying on our principal over the years to reduce our total interest costs.

A fourth element was a benefit offered to employees of Wheaton College. If our children were accepted into Wheaton (or one of the other Christian colleges affiliated with Wheaton) and continued to do well in their classes, the college would pay their tuition for all four years. Furthermore, by the time Diane was ready to enter college, I would have just completed the four years necessary to receive the full benefit! Once again, all the components needed for a solution to our problem had fallen into place. And yet again there was strong evidence, years before this crisis occurred, the Lord had been guiding and providing a way for us to manage it. When we finally grasped this, all we could do was bow our heads and thank God for His love and provision for us. That same day, Ken began the search for a suitable house.

The search didn't take long. Ken found a smaller house in St. Charles that had been newly remodeled and was a little larger than their former apartment. Both Elsie and Emil liked the house, so we completed the purchase and helped them move in and get settled. Brian and Niel mowed their lawn until Emil found a young man in the neighborhood who would do this job, and I contacted a cleaning service to help them with housekeeping. Unfortunately, that arrangement didn't last very long. One of the cleaning ladies was African American, and on her first visit, Emil insulted her badly, even poking her rudely with his cane!

Ken and I knew this was likely to happen again if we tried other cleaning services, so our only other option was for me or Diane to do the weekly cleaning. Since I was in the middle of that first year of teaching, I was already stretched by my responsibilities at home and at work. However, Diane had been hoping to find a part-time job, so when I offered her this job for pay, she accepted it gladly. This was a good solution for everyone. Diane could earn some extra money, and she also was more likely to get along with her grumpy grandpa than someone he didn't know. Elsie was delighted because this gave her opportunity to see Diane more frequently.

This new living situation worked well for a time, until Emil began having difficulty remembering how to get from place to place while driving. One day he set out on an errand and could not find his way back home! He knocked on doors and eventually found a man who let him use his telephone so he could call us to come and rescue him. After that, Emil stopped driving. Since Elsie didn't drive, that meant one of us would need to take them to medical appointments, stores, or run other errands. Fortunately (or should I again say, "by the Lord's provision") by that time, both Diane and Brian had their licenses to drive, so there were four of us who could share that duty. Emil also signed over ownership of his car to Ken so we could keep it at our house and maintain it. That way it would be available for Diane or Brian to use to help their grandparents or for some of their own needs.

A few months after the driving incident, another problem emerged. Emil would get very angry with the boy who delivered their newspapers whenever the paper landed in the yard instead of on the porch. He would fume when a neighbor let his dog run loose and it visited their yard. More seriously, he started getting dreadfully angry with Elsie for no apparent reason, once even threatening to shoot her.

Elsie told Ken about these incidents, and yet again, he had to struggle to keep his frustration in check. Emil had been showing other signs of instability, and Ken knew that he had to find a way to remove that gun safely, legally, and as quickly as possible. He couldn't just walk in and take it because he wasn't physically able to do that nor did he want to expose any of us to potential harm. So he called an attorney who helped him get legal guardianship for his dad; he waited until Emil was not at home, and he and Brian removed the gun and ammunition, taking them immediately to a nearby police station for safekeeping. When Emil learned what Ken had done, he complained bitterly to Elsie, but he never did say anything about it to Ken. Confiscating the gun in this way didn't help Ken's or my own relationship with Emil, but at least it removed a potential source of violence.

In 1980, in the midst of our difficulties with Emil, there were some very positive events. That spring, Diane received notice from Wheaton College that she had been accepted for the fall term. Shortly after that, I received an intriguing letter from my half-sister, Carol, who was then serving in the army and stationed in Germany. While there, she had married another soldier, and she and Marc were both being discharged in two months. Marc's mother owned a villa in southern France, in Biarritz, only three blocks from a very nice beach on the Bay of Biscay. Carol and Marc were planning to stay at that villa for several weeks after their discharge and wanted to know if Ken and I and our family would like to join them there for two or three weeks. We would have to pay for transportation but not for housing and only modestly for food. There was a maid who came in regularly to clean the villa, but Carol and I would have to do the grocery shopping and the cooking during our stay. Since Marc spoke French fluently and was very familiar with the area, shopping and getting around to see things would not be a problem. While there, we could relax at the villa, visit the beach, and take day trips to interesting sites in southern France and northern Spain.

This offer was hard to resist because it gave us a chance to travel abroad—something we hadn't anticipated that we could do. It also appealed to Brian and Niel. Their eagerness to go with us actually made the trip more feasible because they were nearly grown and could help with baggage or difficult physical situations Ken or I might encounter on the trip. Diane didn't want to be away from St. Charles at that time and generously offered to help Elsie and Emil with all their needs while we were gone. The only issues that were still uncertain were how Ken would manage on the long flight to France and how well he could get up and down the stairs to the bedroom we would use in the villa. He was fairly confident he could manage on the airplane because he had successfully taken several flights within the United States to attend academic conferences. Carol also assured us that the stairs to our bedroom had sturdy handrails, so we accepted her invitation.

Consequently, we celebrated Diane's high school graduation in early June, and shortly after, four of us were on our way to France. The villa, the beach, and the countryside in southern France and northern Spain were beautiful. It was really educational to be in a country where English was not the spoken language and where customs and foods were often very different. Carol and I enjoyed experimenting with new foods and recipes and were grateful that Marc was along to interpret and pay the bills when we had to shop for groceries.

Traveling together to see the sights was not as easy as Carol had envisioned. Marc had access to one car, which always remained at the villa, but it was very small and certainly couldn't accommodate six adults. He was able to borrow an additional, larger car from the housekeeper but then had to find a second driver. At that time, anyone with a valid driver's license from the US could legally drive in France. However, Carol's license had expired, Ken and I needed hand controls, and Brian had his license but was seventeen—one year younger than the legal driving age. Fortunately, the local police confirmed that it was still permissible for Brian to drive.

So whenever we went out together, we traveled in a two-car convoy. The country roads that we used for much of that travel were narrow, had many sharp curves, and passed incredibly close to the front doors of houses in smaller towns and villages. Marc and Carol took the lead in the smaller car on these outings, and Marc drove within the speed limits, but since we were not accustomed to taking sharp turns in a very small car or to hearing the tires squeal nearly every time we did it, for a while it felt like we were traveling impossibly fast. We soon learned to grab the hand-holds and brace ourselves when we started around curves. To his credit, Brian adjusted quickly to the stick shift and different driving conditions.

The day trips we took were fascinating. It was amazing to see buildings and churches that were built during the Middle Ages, striking to view the patchwork of small fields and vineyards that dotted the countryside, and surprising to learn that the corn that was so abundant in the fields around us was only used to feed the livestock. To the French, at least at that time and place, corn was considered unfit for human consumption.

When we entered Spain, it was unnerving to see military guards armed with submachine guns at border crossings and at strategic locations within the cities. The areas we visited were in Basque country, and Basque separatists, who didn't want to be a part of Spain, were engaging in systematic acts of violence, often using dynamite to blow up carefully targeted buildings. The Spanish government had sent military guards into the area to try to keep the peace. Marc was well aware of these dangers and made sure to check with his Basque housekeeper to see what areas would be safe to visit on any given day. She evidently knew who to call to get this information!

This trip was especially meaningful for Ken and gave all of us the opportunity to learn a lot more about the French and Spanish people and what it might be like to live in a different culture. In addition to seeing a number of interesting places, it also gave us good opportunities to tell Carol and Marc about our faith and to spend quality time with Brian and Niel at this important stage in their lives.

After we returned from France, I helped Diane gather the supplies she would need that fall for dormitory life. And since she would likely be fully occupied with schoolwork on most of her weekends, I asked Niel to help me with the weekly cleaning for Emil and Elsie. Ken and Brian readily agreed to take them on errands and appointments while Diane was away. With those issues settled, I began preparing for classes.

There was much to be done. Because of personnel changes in our department and my broad background in psychology, I had been responsible for teaching eight different courses in my first four years at Wheaton. My regular courses had been taught four or five times and were well developed, but the extra, "fill-in" courses had been taught only once or twice and still needed work. This need was reflected in some of the student evaluations for those courses.

The fall semester began well, but a few weeks into it, I faced a situation that became very stressful. Assistant professors were eligible to apply for promotion to Associate Professor in their fourth year of teaching so I completed the necessary paperwork and gave it to my department chair. After reading through my application, he told me that he was approving me for reappointment but not for promotion that year because he didn't think my teaching evaluations were as strong or consistent between classes as they needed to be. In addition, the Board of Trustees had also begun using more stringent criteria for promotion. Besides strong evidence of excellence in the classroom, they were also requiring some scholarly presentations and publications and professional recognition from places other than Wheaton. At this early stage of my career, I had little to put down in this latter category other than my attendance at a few professional conferences.

In retrospect, I know my department chair made the right call because he didn't want me to apply unless or until I had credentials that were very likely to be approved by the board. Yet at the time, this news left me feeling very frustrated and anxious. I was anxious because I didn't know what this meant for my future at Wheaton. I was frustrated because I had been working diligently to develop my classes and praying earnestly that I could rightly divide my time between my responsibilities at Wheaton and at home, yet apparently, that wasn't enough. The discrepancy between the board's promotion standards and the priorities I had at that time was also troubling. I believed that my primary responsibility was to teach and wasn't willing to push professional development (e.g., working on research, publications, or presentations) at the expense of class preparation or spending adequate time with my husband and family. Our teens were rapidly transforming into young adults.

Some weeks passed before I learned that I could, without penalty, successfully apply for promotion a year or two later after building up the required credentials. That information brought a sense of relief, but the need to apply "late" still chafed. It also challenged some of my expectations and assumptions. Consequently, I went through a period of frustration and questioning, which God used to teach *me* some new ways of thinking.

In graduate school, I had become accustomed to getting very high grades and comparing myself to other students to build up self-confidence and self-esteem. However, the need to apply for promotion later than expected undermined my confidence and even prompted me to question whether I was actually capable of teaching at Wheaton's standards! A quick review of the unlikely circumstances that had brought me to Wheaton reassured me that this fear was bogus. It was clearly God who had opened this door of opportunity, and that meant I had the requisite ability because God doesn't make mistakes! Further thought also helped me recognized the folly of comparing myself with others (in this case, my colleagues). In reality, all of us had all been called to our work at Wheaton and God had equipped each of us with the particular abilities we needed for our different tasks. Moreover, we were there to be working together toward the common goal of educating our students and equipping them to live obedient and effective lives as Christians—not to be comparing or competing with one another. The only thing I really needed to be concerned about was how well I was measuring up to the calling God had given me!

I had also wrongly assumed that if I had the ability to teach well, it shouldn't take a lot of time or effort to learn to do so. However, a bit of reflection revealed that this wasn't necessarily true. There were many biblical accounts of believers who had to struggle greatly to remain faithful and fulfill God's calling for them. Moreover, their struggles were not meaningless. God used those difficulties to teach them perseverance, patience, and a greater dependence on and trust in Him. Therefore, I couldn't just assume that my calling to teach would be any different.

As I had opportunity to observe effective teachers, I did learn that many of the characteristics that I originally thought were important (e.g., an impressive appearance, a commanding classroom presence, a strong resonant voice, etc.) were not prerequisites either. The best teachers were those who successfully engaged student interest and enthusiasm in what they were teaching and helped students see its meaning, relevance, and application to their own lives. In fact, teaching seemed to be most effective when students were not attending to the personal characteristics of the teacher at all but were totally absorbed with what he or she was communicating. Over time and with effort, I gradually acquired this skill myself. What delighted me most were the opportunities to focus student attention on the mysterious and majestic God who created our remarkable world and the astonishing perceptual, mental, and physical capabilities He built into human beings!

Shortly before the promotion issue surfaced, Brian, who was just a year behind Diane in high school, also applied for admission to Wheaton College. In the spring of 1981, he was accepted at Wheaton and entered a "three-two" cooperative program in

Electrical Engineering, attending Wheaton for three years and the University of Illinois for two more, earning a bachelor's degree from both. Since both Brian and Diane lived on campus that year, Ken, Niel, and I shared the responsibility of helping Elsie and Emil.

After the fall term ended that year, we celebrated Christmas together with Ken's parents as we had done for so many years before. However, just ten days later, in early January, we received an urgent telephone call from Elsie. She had called an ambulance for Emil because it appeared that he was having a heart attack. We drove to their house as quickly as possible, but Emil died before we could get there. He lost consciousness before the ambulance arrived, and the paramedics were not able to revive him.

Emil was in his eighties, but the suddenness of his death still caught us off guard. Our sorrow was compounded by the fact that he had never surrendered his life to Jesus. Emil had known the way of salvation from childhood and had told Elsie that he did believe that God was real. However, he had also declared that he was going to live life his own way. Emil's funeral was a very somber event. It didn't help that the day was dark and bitterly cold, and only a few of us were gathered at our small church. The emptiness in the church echoed the emptiness and futility of a life lived apart from Christ, and the sullen darkness of the day kept reminding us of the terrible darkness Emil had entered.

Our most immediate concern after Emil's death was for Elsie's well-being. She came to live with us for a while but decided she wanted to go back to her home. At first we were reluctant but chose to honor her wishes, resolving to stay in close contact. It helped that Niel was driving close by where she lived every weekday on his way to and from high school. He stopped there often on his way home to check on his grandmother, to see if she needed anything, and just to visit with her for a while. Ken and I also called, visited, and had her over for meals as often as possible.

This arrangement worked reasonably well for a couple of months. However, one afternoon, right after Niel had left school for home, he felt a strong, unexplainable urge to turn down the street where Elsie lived to check on her. He hadn't planned to stop that afternoon, but a growing sense of uneasiness and urgency compelled him to do so. He pulled into the driveway, walked hurriedly to the front door, and knocked. There was no answer! The door was unlocked, so he pushed it open. Elsie was sitting in her favorite chair, but he could tell immediately that something was wrong. She acknowledged his presence by her facial expression and by moving one hand a little, but she couldn't talk and couldn't get up by herself! Niel quickly called an ambulance.

Elsie had suffered another serious stroke. She was in the hospital for about a month but did not recover much function. She was not able to sit up or turn over in bed by herself or to eat and swallow normally. Many times she recognized us and could speak one or two words in answer to our questions, but there were also a few times when she was completely unresponsive. Her doctor finally confirmed what we suspected, that she needed twenty-four-hour, skilled nursing care, and our only option was to move her to a nursing home. Having to do this was very difficult because we didn't know how much she was aware of or how much she might be suffering, and we certainly didn't want her to feel alone.

Elsie was in the this facility nearly a year and a half, and during that time, her health slowly declined. One of my greatest concerns was whether her faith could sustain her in such difficult circumstances. We brought Elsie her radio so she could listen to Christian broadcasting from WMBI in Chicago, as she had done for many years at home, and I would read portions of the Bible to her on visits when she seemed alert, but I had no way of knowing how she was coping. Finally, on one visit when she was more alert and responsive than usual, I simply asked her, "Mom, how is your faith in God?" With little hesitation, a hint of a smile and surprising strength and conviction, she stated, "It is fine." That was an encouragement we all needed. Evidently her strong faith had also witnessed to several of the workers who cared for her regularly, even though her verbal communication was so limited. Independently two different caregivers asked me if Elsie was a Christian—simply because her behavior.

Elsie struggled on until the middle of October and then left this life. Her funeral service and burial contrasted markedly with Emil's. We were fully assured that she was now in Heaven and that one day we would be with her again. The day was also warm and sunny and the trees were ablaze with celebratory color. In addition, our sorrow at Elsie's departure was mingled with relief and even joy—relief because her suffering was over and joy because she had triumphantly finished the race, keeping her faith and her witness in spite of all the daunting obstacles in her path.

The Christmas following her death was subdued because neither Elsie nor Emil were with us and there were now only the five of us around the table for Christmas dinner. In addition, on that day, it wasn't clear what Christmas dinners might look like in the near future because our fledglings were clearly in the process of leaving the nest. We didn't know who they might marry or where they might live and whether we would even be together very often on such occasions. Fortunately, these concerns never became a serious issue because Diane, Brian, and Niel all chose to remain in the same area, at least in part because they realized that we would probably need their help as we grew older! As a result, 1984 actually marked the beginning of an extended period of deep gratification and unanticipated joy for all of us.

At this point, my obligations at home and at work became much more manageable. We were able to sell Elsie and Emil's house fairly quickly, so our responsibilities there were completed. Since Diane and Brian were living on campus most of the year and only three of us remained at home, my housekeeping and cooking duties were significantly reduced. Wheaton College had also switched from quarters to semesters, and I was teaching the same four or five classes every year, so I finally had time to devote to professional development. I also felt much more settled and confident in my career because I had been promoted to Associate Professor the year before and received tenure early in 1984. As an added blessing, within that same time frame, Ken was promoted to Senior Scientist at Argonne, which was equivalent to being a Full Professor in the university system. Looking back at all the twists, turns, and obstacles in our lives, both of us had to marvel at how the Lord had helped us to attain what had seemed so unattainable.

My reduced workload allowed me to have more time with Ken than we had had since getting married. Thanks to the Lord's relentless shaping in the earlier years of our marriage, our relationship was strong and deep, and we counted each other as best friends and confidants as well as husband and wife. Since we still shared a keen interest in seeing new places and both of us were still relatively able, physically, we decided to search for a way that just the two of us could travel comfortably on extended trips. We still enjoyed camping but couldn't manage the trailer by ourselves, so we started researching smaller motorhomes. If we could find one we could modify, we could use it for sight-seeing during the day and simply park it in a campsite at night.

After quite a bit of searching, we did locate a twenty-three footer that could be equipped with hand controls and met all but one of our other needs. Its only drawback was the first high step into the vehicle. Portable steps were not feasible, but after some thought, we realized that if that first steel step, which was sturdy and fairly large, could somehow be transformed into a miniature lift, this motorhome would work. Eventually we located an innovative mechanic who was willing to take on this unique project. Using small hydraulic cylinders, an electric motor, and some extra parts, he transformed the first step into a platform that could be lowered to the ground with the press of a switch. Ken could then step onto the platform and use the switch to lift the platform back to its original position. The second and third steps into the motorhome were not as high as the first, and there were handrails on both sides, so Ken was able to climb these in his usual manner.

It took a bit of practice to get used to driving this larger vehicle, but with it we were able to refuel and perform all the other functions needed by ourselves. Over the eight years we used it, we traveled to both the east and west coasts, down into Florida, and up into Canada, enjoying many national parks and monuments along the way. We also utilized the motorhome for family outings and day trips when our family started to expand. And we counted every trip as an added blessing from the Lord.

The most significant and exciting change that occurred during this period began in 1984 when our family stopped shrinking and began to grow! That May, Diane graduated from Wheaton, moved home for a time, and found employment at a Christian publishing company. That June, Niel graduated from high school, married Regina, found a job, and moved out to start his own family. The next May, Diane married Gary, a Christian man she had been dating for several years, and they moved into an apartment just a few miles away. Over the next seven years, we were blessed with five new grandchildren! Brian graduated from Wheaton and the University of Illinois but didn't marry right away. When he did, he and Amy added three more grandchildren. By that time our family had increased from five to sixteen!

It is an understatement to say that this was an amazing, fulfilling, and wonderful period in our lives. We had not anticipated how significantly our lives would be changed and enriched by the addition of all these new family members or the joy of having grandchildren, being able to interact with them often, and watching them grow and develop. It seemed that there were always baby showers and birthdays to plan for and attend. Holidays like Easter, Thanksgiving, and Christmas were all enriched immensely. Lest I leave you with the wrong impression, our family did have its share of difficulties and struggles during this period, but on the whole, it was an incredible time of blessing and growth.

Chapter 12

Round Two with an Old Adversary

I t was in the midst of those delightful years of family growth, grandchildren, new opportunities to travel, and increased fulfillment at work that our old nemesis, polio, reappeared in a new manifestation, once more threatening to totally disrupt our lives. We were watching the nightly news when we heard that physicians had identified a new disorder called "Post-Polio Syndrome." This was primarily afflicting people who had contracted polio thirty-five to forty years previously and had also recovered a significant amount of function. However, they were now experiencing new and debilitating weaknesses, paralysis, and pain. This was occurring not only in muscles that were originally weakened by the virus but also in muscles that hadn't appeared to have been affected at all. These changes were forcing victims to rely on canes, crutches, braces, or wheelchairs to get around and, in some cases, on ventilators to help them breathe!

There was no evidence that the polio virus had revived and was inflicting new damage but, rather, that motor neurons that had branched extensively after the initial infection were either dying early (possibly because they were chronically overworked) or were withdrawing from the extra connections they had made in order to survive. The resulting loss of innervation was apparently causing the renewed muscle weakness and paralysis.

This report alarmed both of us but was particularly upsetting to me. It was distressing to think that I might be confined to a wheelchair again or even to imagine how we could continue to function if that were to happen. We quickly reviewed our own physical status. I hadn't observed any new weaknesses, but Ken, who had polio thirty-six years earlier, definitely was. For several years, he had noticed slowly increasing pain and weakness in his shoulders, arms, and wrists, which was particularly evident when he used his braces and crutches to walk. However, Ken didn't believe these problems were necessarily due to post-polio syndrome because, to his knowledge, polio hadn't affected his arms or shoulders. He thought it more likely that his current problems were due to many years of abuse, forcing the muscles and joints in his arms and shoulders to work vigorously and unnaturally to help him walk on crutches and braces and to push his wheelchair. I was pretty sure I was seeing some increased weaknesses in his back and abdominal muscles because of subtle changes in his posture and balance. However, these changes seemed minor, so I didn't mention them. Truth be told, I was so apprehensive about the damage that post-polio syndrome might inflict upon us, I was hoping against hope that if we didn't acknowledge its presence, it might just go away.

Ken continued to search for more information but remained calm about his own situation. He had already accepted the fact that he wasn't going to be able to use his crutches and braces on a daily basis much longer. This wasn't a problem at home because he was already doing all that was needed from his wheelchair. However, it did create a significant problem at Argonne. He considered the possibility of using his wheelchair at work because his office and the building in which it was located were accessible. However, with his shoulder problems, it would have been very difficult and painful for him to get his wheelchair in and out of the car every day by himself. The only way he could continue to work would be to purchase a van equipped with a lift, and that would be very expensive.

Since Ken had worked for more than thirty years and had also been experiencing a lot of general fatigue as well as pain in his arms and shoulders, he asked if I would object if he took early retirement. This was not a problem financially. Ken would receive ample monthly annuity income, he had built up substantial savings, we had no debts, and my position at Wheaton was secure. Ken had wide and varied interests, so I wasn't concerned that he would be bored. Besides that, I knew that if my very disciplined, responsible, and hard-working husband wanted to retire early, he undoubtedly had some very strong reasons for doing so. I offered Ken my whole-hearted support, and he retired in 1989, at the age of fifty-eight.

Ken's physical difficulties and his retirement didn't alter our lifestyle for quite a while. In retirement, he used the crutches and braces much less frequently and his shoulders improved, enabling him to continue to use the crutches for church and other outings. I also learned how to get his lightweight wheelchair in and out of the motorhome and our car so he could use it at many of our destinations. This also allowed us to continue to take trips in the motorhome.

Changes in my own physical ability started appearing very gradually a year or so after Ken retired. At that time, we used to go for "walks" on bike paths or on our development roads to get some exercise and fresh air. (I walked, Ken pushed himself along in his wheelchair.) Over time, I started feeling fatigued on these outings, so I started using my crutch and, later, my own new wheelchair.

As time passed, I also began to have serious bouts of pain in my lower back, along with muscle fatigue and unusual problems with digestion. These problems persisted and grew worse, so I eventually went to the Mayo Clinic for diagnosis. The doctors at Mayo concluded that the problems with digestion were probably related to long-standing food allergies and sensitivities and that the back pain was being caused by *weakening back muscles*. That latter diagnosis helped me understand a puzzling incident that had taken place shortly before I visited Mayo. Diane and I were standing and talking when she paused, started looking at me rather oddly, stepped back, and then exclaimed, "Mom, you are standing crooked!" I was leaning slightly forward and toward my right from my waist even though it felt to me like I was standing straight. The only way I could verify what she saw was to see it for myself in a full-length mirror.

After the trip to Mayo, the back pain continued, I had more tests, and an orthopedist discovered an arthritic spur on a disc in my spine that he thought might be causing the pain. I had microsurgery that removed the spur, but that didn't help. Finally I made an appointment with a physiatrist at a nearby rehabilitation hospital who knew about polio and post-polio syndrome. He confirmed what I feared the most. The increasing weakness and pain in the muscles in my lower back, abdomen, and quadriceps in both legs were most likely an indication of post-polio syndrome since these were muscles that had been most severely affected by the virus thirty-five years earlier. He prescribed a back support, which helped alleviate the back pain, and warned me not to try to build more strength in weakening muscles by vigorous exercise. Doing so might worsen my condition quickly and permanently. (Overtaxing neurons that were already overworked would hasten their death.) I did need moderate exercise, but if I experienced unusual pain or fatigue, I needed to stop immediately and rest.

Even after that appointment, I was still reluctant to accept the diagnosis because its implications were overwhelming. If I couldn't walk or stand without support, could I continue to teach effectively? If I were confined to a wheelchair, how could we continue to function independently, especially since Ken was now less able? Then I realized that if I did become wheelchair bound, we would either have to move to more accessible quarters or make huge modifications in our house! My heart sank.

This whole scenario seemed so incomprehensible and unnecessary that I couldn't see how it could possibly be in the Lord's will. I asked friends at the Baptist church I was then attending to pray that I would not be further disabled. Later I also asked my pastor for special prayer. In a private session with all three pastors, after a time of confession and repentance, my senior pastor anointed my head with oil (as instructed in James 5:14-15) and all three pastors prayed for my physical healing. That calmed my soul, but it didn't change what was happening in my body. As I would understand later, in this case the Lord's answer was "no" for my good and His greater glory. He was letting nature take its course, even though that did mean that I would be using a wheelchair for the rest of my life!

It was really difficult for me to relinquish my will in this matter and to ask, instead, that the Lord's will be done. But I finally did so, and shortly after that I realized that instead of being resentful, I should be very grateful. My initial recovery from polio had given me thirty-five years of walking and fairly normal function. If God had not built in this ability to recover, I would have been confined to a wheelchair for that entire time and my life would have been very different. That thirty-five years of restored function made it feasible to marry Ken and enabled us to live independently. It had also given us the ability to acquire and maintain a home, to raise a family, to get an education, and for me to teach and serve at Wheaton College!

When I finally faced reality, Ken and I began assessing our situation and working on possible solutions. The changes we needed to make were daunting. Our bedroom was too small to allow two wheelchairs to maneuver easily between the bed and the other furniture. Our bathtub was becoming difficult for Ken to enter and exit safely because of the weakness and pain in his shoulders. The bathroom was too small—just large enough to allow one wheelchair to enter, pull forward to the lavatory, toilet, or tub and then to back out. The kitchen was becoming unusable because the countertops, sink, and range top, which were positioned at standard heights, reached right to the top of my shoulders when I was seated in the wheelchair. In addition, the ramp leading from the garage into the house was far too steep.

Transportation was another serious issue. My increasing weakness meant that we weren't going to be able to use the motorhome much longer or, for that matter, even to be able to travel together in one car! It would be difficult to stow two wheelchairs in either car and would eventually become impossible for me to get them in or out by myself.

The third area of concern was how I could continue to function effectively at Wheaton. This was the most immediate challenge, but fortunately, it was also the easiest to deal with. At first I used a wheelchair to get to and from the car and my office, walked the short distance to the classroom using my crutch, and sat on a high stool to teach. Most of my classes were already being taught in seminar rooms with the students seated around a table, so I was able to continue to teach much as I had before. As my difficulties with standing and walking increased, I gradually started teaching and getting from place to place entirely in my wheelchair. My earlier fears that teaching from a wheelchair might decrease my effectiveness also proved to be unfounded. I'm not sure how this happened, but if anything, teaching from the wheelchair, without being concerned or apologetic about it, seemed to give me as much or even a little more credibility with the students. The only significant change I had to make was to discontinue lecturing in Introductory Psychology, and that was simply because the stage in the lecture hall was not wheelchair accessible.

Fortunately (and once again, most assuredly by the Lord's provision) during the two years in which Ken and I sought and implemented solutions for our housing and transportation problems, my strength declined slowly enough to allow us to do what we needed. Since we were still able to travel together in a car, we tackled the housing issue first. We needed a completely new kitchen, a larger bathroom with accessible bathing facilities, a larger master bedroom, and a larger garage with a longer and wider ramp. At that point, our house was thirty years old, so it was also time to replace the roofing, windows, and siding. After exploring our options, it appeared that our best choice was to remodel and enlarge our existing house.

I was able to find an excellent architect and a builder who were both Christians by making inquiries at the college. Before we met with the architect, Ken and I spent a lot of time working out the needed modifications, making scaled drawings of our furniture and wheelchairs, and moving these about in floor plans drawn to the same scale so we could estimate how large various rooms would need to be. Since our family was still growing, we also wanted to expand the dining/family room area to accommodate larger gatherings. Thankfully, our architect was able to pull all of our requirements together into an esthetically pleasing and functional plan. This doubled the size of our house. Only the original bathroom and bedrooms remained the same.

When we met with our builder, Todd Walker, in the summer of 1993, we had to decide when to do the remodeling and where we would live while it was being done. Todd scheduled the work for the spring and summer of 1994. I asked him to start in early May, when classes at Wheaton were ending, and to finish by the end of August so I would have a few days to get the house in order before starting to teach in the fall. Amazingly, he accomplished the complete remodeling job with a few days to spare, even though that often meant having large numbers of his crew and subcontractors working on the job at the same time.

We decided to stay in our home during the remodeling, living mostly in our bedroom, using a second bedroom to store our extra furniture and the smaller bedroom partly for storage and partly as a small study so I could continue to prepare for classes. We could still use the bathroom, but our kitchen was being demolished so we used the kitchen and dining area in the motorhome for meals. Todd built a temporary ramp for our front stoop so Ken and I could get out the front door in our wheelchairs and push across the lawn to the motorhome, which was parked nearby. Once there, Ken used his braces and crutches to get in and maneuver inside. I had to walk, occasionally supporting myself with my arms, and to sit on a high stool to prepare our meals and wash dishes. Managing in these conditions was not easy, but our conviction that the Lord was guiding this process gave us the courage and strength to do it.

We did encounter some substantial design challenges, particularly in the kitchen and bathroom. In the kitchen, I needed a workspace, sink, and cooktop that would be low enough to use for food preparation while seated in the wheelchair but also high enough and with enough clearance underneath to allow me to pull in under these in the wheelchair. Figuring out where to place these elements was relatively easy, but finding a safe cooktop was not. Since I would be seated while using it and reaching over burners without much clearance, a gas cooktop with open flames would be hazardous as would a ceramic cooktop, which would retain a lot of heat. The safest alternative, fairly innovative at the time, was an induction cooktop. The "burners" on these cooktops used rapidly alternating magnetic fields to induce heat in pans made of iron or steel (to which magnets are attracted), and the pans transferred that heat to their contents. Since the cooktop was heated only by the pot or pan, it remained relatively cool.

Another issue we faced in the kitchen was building in sufficient storage. I needed ample lower cabinet space because I didn't know how long I would be able to stand up and reach into upper cabinets. Yet much of the space in the kitchen that would normally be used for lower cabinets was needed to provide access for wheelchairs. We did plan to include upper cabinets regardless of any future difficulties I might be facing, so I knew these would give me adequate storage space at least for a while. However, Todd came up with the idea of adding an L-shaped row of lower (and some upper) cabinets, topped with a solid-surface counter, along the western and northern boundaries of the kitchen. This not only provided an attractive and functional partition between the kitchen and the rest of the great room but also provided space for additional lower cabinets.

That feature solved another problem as well. I had requested double ovens. However, for both to be accessible, they needed to be side by side rather than one on top of the other. The long partition designed to house extra lower cabinets also provided a convenient place for the ovens. Placing them there did require the countertop to be thirty-four inches high, and that was too high for me to use as a work surface. However, I could still reach to put things on it, and it was perfect for serving buffet dinners. In addition, the counter's near-normal height increased the storage capacity of the cabinets underneath and helped to camouflage the shortness of the cabinets and workspaces along the kitchen walls.

Designing this kitchen so it was functional and still looked attractive was another challenge. The kitchen was part of the great room, and the entire room had a high cathedral ceiling. Both its east and west walls rose to a height of sixteen feet at their centers. The west wall was balanced by wide, centered, sliding glass doors with tall cathedral windows positioned above them. However, the inner kitchen cabinets and workspaces were located along parts of the east and south walls, so the question was how to keep the upper and lower cabinets, which were to be placed several inches lower than normal, from looking too short, even "squashed" compared to the sixteen-foot peak in the east wall right behind them.

Todd suggested that we could minimize this problem by installing the upper cabinets beneath a soffit, placed with its top at a height of eight feet. However, to reach to the tops of the upper cabinets, the soffit would also have to be several inches taller than normal, making it seem disproportionately large. At that point, it occurred to me that we could probably camouflage the soffit's height by breaking it up with a prominent horizontal wallpaper border running along its middle and a contrasting crown molding extending horizontally along its top. (That trick worked well.) The soffit also provided a natural place for much-needed task lighting over the work areas. After construction was finished, I was able to make the kitchen appear even taller, relative to the wall behind it, by placing a variety of stately bird cages on top of the soffit.

Because the heights of our cabinets were not standard, Todd suggested that we order custom cabinets from an Amish company with whom he had worked before. We chose to have the cabinets made of hickory, because its grain was attractive and the hard wood would resist unintended dents and scrapes from our wheelchairs. When the cabinets and kitchen counters were delivered, we were very impressed with the beauty and precision with which they were built. Remarkably, each premade piece fit perfectly into place, in spite of all the adaptations and unusual requirements in the floor plan.

Compared to the kitchen, designing an accessible bathroom was relatively easy. This room was large because we wanted to be able to utilize that space at the same time in our wheelchairs. The roll-in shower had a built-in bench and a shower head that could be positioned at different heights or held in one's hand. There was also a built-in whirlpool bathtub. The top of the enclosure around the tub was almost level with the top of the tub and extended out far enough on two sides to provide a flat surface on which to sit or transfer to from a wheelchair. We found a simple, water-powered lift, made in Germany, that solved the problem of how to get down in and up out of that deep tub. The room also included two wheelchair-accessible vanities with mirrored cabinets above them.

Construction commenced in the spring of 1994 and proceeded on schedule with only minor glitches. Many on Todd's construction crew were Christians and were enthusiastic about our unique project. It was a pleasure to get to know and interact with them. When construction was completed, Ken and I were delighted with the results. Once again, we were very thankful that God had helped us find a way and to have the resources not only to modify our home so it worked for two wheelchair users but also to make it even better and more attractive than it had been before. Once more we were reminded that nothing is impossible with God and that He is always able to do far more than all we could ask or imagine (Ephesians 3:20-21).

After the house was completed, Ken and I immediately started working on our transportation needs. With many fond memories and some sadness, we sold our motorhome the following spring. We knew that it was possible to equip vans with hand controls and wheelchair lifts. What we did not know was whether it would be possible to customize a van for two wheelchair users in a way that would allow either of us to drive and the other to ride as a passenger. After quite a bit of prayer and searching, we discovered a small company that did accessible van conversions, and their designer was able to devise a workable plan.

The crew started with a new, full-sized Ford van that came with a driver's and passenger's seat plus a single bench seat in the back. They removed the passenger's seat and modified the driver's seat so it could be moved back and forth from the steering wheel by about two feet, adjusted in height by about eight inches, and swiveled a full 120 degrees, all by pressing switches. This capability allowed Ken to position the seat so he could transfer directly into it from his wheelchair using just his arms. The space normally occupied by a passenger seat was empty except for a small steel box on the floor that locked Ken's wheelchair in place. The rest of the interior was left open to allow as much room as possible for us to maneuver in our chairs. The conversion work took some time, but we finally drove out to the shop to pick up our van early in December of 1995.

Going places together in the van was not easy, but it was possible, and for that we were very grateful. When we traveled together, we did have to follow a definite protocol. One of us would start the sequence by using a four-function remote that swung open the two van doors, unfolded a three-panel lift, swung the lift from a vertical to a horizontal position, and then lowered the lift to the garage floor. I would use the lift first, enter, and push to the back of the van in my wheelchair. I then stood, folded my chair, and belted it in. If Ken planned to drive, I would sit in the back seat and wait for him to lower the lift, enter, and transfer to the driver's seat. I would then walk forward, supporting myself as needed with my arms, sit in his wheelchair and pull it into the locking device on the passenger's side. While Ken used interior controls to fold the lift and shut the doors, I checked the chair lock and fastened my seat belt. After that, we were finally ready to depart. When I drove, the procedure was simpler. After stowing my chair, I would simply walk forward and wait in the driver's seat while Ken to entered and pulled his wheelchair into the locking mechanism.

I should note that this particular protocol and, more generally, our ability to use the van together at all did depend upon my continuing ability to walk with some support for short distances and to maneuver our wheelchairs inside the van. Getting the van set up on the assumption that I would continue to be able to do these things seemed risky, but there was no other way to make it work! In this case, we did everything we could to prepare for future eventualities but then simply had to trust that the Lord was guiding the process so that would be enough. In retrospect, that guidance was very evident. Against the odds, I retained the physical ability to do the things that were necessary for the thirteen years they were needed and even well beyond!

Looking back, it was also clearly in the Lord's timing that we were able to finish the remodeling, get the van, and learn how to use it when we did. Just four months later, Ken faced a major health crisis that would have been impossible for us to manage without these modifications. Actually, Ken was not feeling quite himself when we picked up the van in December. He was struggling with increased muscle pain, fatigue, and drowsiness. Since he was also having difficulty sleeping, he just assumed that his poor sleep was causing him to feel fatigued and drowsy during the day. By early April of 1996, Ken's fatigue became noticeably worse. He would feel tired and out of breath after just pushing his wheelchair out to the mailbox and then back up the ramp and into the house.

Ken was being treated for high blood pressure at the time, and at his next scheduled appointment, he told his cardiologist about his new problems. Dr. Wang immediately ran an electrocardiogram, and what he saw in the tracings clearly alarmed him. Ken was at high risk for a heart attack, and Dr. Wang wanted him to go directly to the hospital to be admitted for observation and testing. Ken had to persuade his doctor to let him drive home to pick me up so I could then drive him to the hospital. When Ken came home from that appointment and told me the news, I was stunned and predictably upset even though he remained calm. We shared a brief time of prayer, hastily gathered a few necessities, and headed straight for the hospital. Ken was admitted on a Wednesday afternoon, but his doctor postponed the angiogram until the following Wednesday when he knew that a particular cardiac surgeon could be there to assist him.

Very early on the morning of that test, our adult children and two of their spouses gathered with me in Ken's room and we prayed together for his recovery and well-being. About an hour later, we learned that Ken had serious blockages in several coronary arteries and that the doctors were proceeding with surgery. After that, time seemed to crawl. It helped that three of our grandkids were with us from the start. Brian's wife, Amy, came later with her toddler and six-month-old baby. Keeping these little ones occupied and quiet was a welcome distraction, and having all of our family there provided incredible support and encouragement for me.

Time kept passing with no additional information, and then, around one o'clock in the afternoon, we learned that Ken's procedure had taken five hours and that he had had open-heart, quadruple-bypass surgery. When we were finally able to see him late that afternoon, he was very pale, was unaware of our presence, and was breathing with the aid of a ventilator. Diane accompanied me home that evening, and I was composed until I wheeled through the utility room and saw some of Ken's clothes among the piles of laundry that I had sorted but hadn't finished laundering. It suddenly flashed through my mind that Ken might never be back home to wear those clothes again, and I started sobbing uncontrollably. But then a very unexpected thing happened! Just as suddenly and very unmistakably, I was filled with a remarkable sense of peace and a deep assurance that Ken was going to recover from this crisis. My tears stopped midstream, and instead of being filled with fear and sorrow, I was filled with joy and thanksgiving! This was an amazing and inexplicable gift! I knew that many friends at Wheaton College and at our church were praying for us. I could only conclude that God had heard and that He was answering.

Even more remarkably, that peace and assurance stayed with me the next several weeks as I juggled the responsibilities of finishing the semester, keeping up with work at home, and visiting the hospital to encourage Ken as he struggled to recover. His heart surgery had gone well, but it was initially very difficult for him to breathe without the ventilator. It was three days before the ventilator could be removed, and Ken needed additional oxygen for several days. Later we were informed that Ken's diaphragm had been seriously damaged *before* the operation, most likely by the polio virus or its late aftereffects.

After getting off the ventilator, Ken started reacting badly to some of his medications. The fact that he couldn't get up and walk led to additional complications. Fifteen days after surgery, he was transferred to a rehabilitation hospital to continue to recover, and he stayed there ten more days before he could come home. Fortunately, by that time I finished my work at Wheaton, so I could be with him continuously and drive him to various appointments. By fall, Ken was much better; however, it took him a full year to recover completely.

Although this crisis had been very difficult and painful for Ken, we had much to be thankful for. We were grateful that this emergency did not occur while we were in the midst of remodeling or before we had the van. It would have been impossible for us to manage by ourselves without that vehicle. We were also very thankful that Ken's heart condition was discovered before he had a heart attack. If he had suffered a major heart attack with a seriously compromised diaphragm, it was unlikely that he would have recovered.

Ken's close brush with death and difficult recovery did help him to grow spiritually. A couple of months into recovery, he was more relaxed and less easily irritated than I ever remembered. Soon after, Ken told me that he had finally been able to forgive his dad completely and had asked for God's forgiveness for holding on to his anger and resentment for so long. A few days after that, Ken announced that he wanted to become a full-fledged member of the Baptist church we attended! That might not seem like a big thing, but for Ken, at that time, it really was.

One of the obstacles to his membership at First Baptist was the requirement of baptism by water immersion. I had been baptized at age twelve and was therefore able to transfer my membership directly from the Covenant church without a problem. However, Ken had not been baptized as an adult, and as an adult, water immersion was not really feasible because of his physical disability. Ken disliked doing anything that called more attention to his physical condition or that might cause others to feel awkward. Moreover, he was convinced that he would appear to be more able if he were standing or walking around with his crutches rather than sitting in a wheelchair. That was a legitimate concern when he first began to work at Argonne in the late 1950s. At that time, he had to do everything he could to convince his supervisor and colleagues that a person with serious physical disabilities could be as capable and productive as an able-bodied worker. This belief also persuaded Ken to keep using his crutches and braces at Argonne even when it would have much easier on his shoulders and arms to use a wheelchair.

Because of these convictions and perhaps partly out of pride, when Ken could no longer use his the crutches and braces, he chose to stop attending church rather than to go there in his wheelchair. Furthermore, he didn't attend for many months. Thus, Ken's new determination to join the church indicated that his perspective had shifted dramatically. He was now willing to do whatever might be necessary to be right with God, even if that put his disability on full display.

Pastor Brian was flexible and decided that the best way to conduct Ken's baptism was to sprinkle him liberally with water, explaining the reasons for this exception to the congregation just before the ceremony. Before his baptism, Ken courageously pushed himself out in front of the congregation in his wheelchair, picked up a microphone, and testified unflinchingly to his lifelong love and trust in Jesus Christ. Even though Ken was probably not aware of it, the fact that he was in a wheelchair and had obviously faced unusual adversity in his life made his testimony even more compelling and credible. That day God's power was clearly on display in Ken's weakness (see second Corinthians 12:9).

Chapter 13

Amazing Grace

One day, not long after his baptism, Ken asked whether I had started thinking about retirement or how I might like to use the extra time that would provide. I was fifty-six at the time, and I think he also wanted to remind me that I could retire early, like he had, if I wanted to. The thought was momentarily appealing because working full time was becoming more tiring. However, teaching was still very meaningful and rewarding, so I didn't anticipate retiring any time soon. Nevertheless, Ken's suggestion that I start planning ahead for it was wise.

As I considered how to use leisure time, my first thought was traveling. However, by that time, we both knew that our decreased physical abilities would make traveling much more difficult, so that was not something we would try very often. My next thought was gardening. Except for maintaining some landscaping and a few pots of flowers, this was something I had discontinued shortly after I started teaching. I had enjoyed gardening immensely. However, when I tried to imagine how I could manage this from a wheelchair, my budding enthusiasm began to wilt. Suddenly gardening just didn't seem that feasible either. Still, I had learned from experience not to jump to hasty conclusions about what I could or could not do. Over the years, the Lord had helped both of us find ways to accomplish many things that at first had seemed impossible.

So instead of just dismissing the idea, I started thinking about gardening tasks I could still carry out. Many of the muscles in my legs and back were still fairly strong, as were my arms and shoulders. I could stand and bend over for two or three minutes with a little support from one arm. On paved surfaces like roads or sidewalks, I could propel myself in the wheelchair using just my legs and feet, leaving my hands free to carry items or to push a lightweight cart. I could also pull weeds, break ground, cultivate, plant seeds, and prune while sitting in the wheelchair.

What would I not be able to do? At that time, my greatest challenge was simply getting to and from the beds that needed tending. Pushing the wheelchair through grass to reach the beds strained my arms and shoulders. Furthermore, using both hands to push made it difficult to transport tools, containers, or anything else. In an "aha" moment, I suddenly realized that if I had paved walkways everywhere I needed to go, I could tend a lot of plants myself!

In fact, placing beds between the house and a paved walkway would offer many benefits. Walkways would keep perennials or shrubs in bounds and keep grass and weeds out and create natural mowing strips. If the walkways were wide enough to allow me to turn around and work at different angles in my wheelchair, the beds were relatively narrow, and I used smaller shrubs and perennials, I could keep my wheelchair on the walkway (and out of the dirt) and reach into the beds to weed and tend the plants. Furthermore, if the walkway went partly or even completely around the house and deck, I could have many accessible beds in both sun and shade. Those beds would also be a natural setting for flowers and other landscaping.

When I drew these plans to scale around the layout of our house and deck, I also noticed that there were places where it would be beneficial to widen parts of the pathway or connect it to paved terraces. On the west side of the house, two such terraces could connect with the two ramps from the deck, making the deck more accessible from outside. Those terraces would also provide more outdoor space that we could utilize in our wheelchairs.

I wanted a vegetable garden, and the idea of inserting terraces as part of the walkway suggested a way to create one. We had a large, sunny, level space for the garden right next to the south side of our house. Placing the inner edge of a terrace three feet away from the foundation would leave space for larger plants like tomatoes, peppers, and zucchini. Adding four parallel raised beds in the middle of the terrace, which could be tended from either side, would provide easily accessed spaces for shorter crops like carrots, green beans, lettuce, etc. In addition, a four-foot fence around the entire garden would not only provide protection from rabbits and deer but also create spaces for more beds. Simply leaving a one-foot gap between the outer edge of the paving and the fence, I could use this space for vining crops like cucumbers, melons, squash, and pole beans, which could be trained to grow up on the fence.

I spent many leisure hours refining these plans, adding some additional features, and searching through articles and catalogues for suitable shrubs and perennials. Early on, I asked Ken if he would like to join me in the planning. He was interested and gave me valuable feedback whenever I requested it, but he also preferred to let me do the planning. I was the avid gardener and also the one who would have to do most of the gardening.

Ken did get a little nervous when the project began to grow (and he probably had some second thoughts about encouraging me to start thinking about leisure activities). However, his main concerns were the cost of the project and whether I was taking on more than I could handle physically. Still, Ken's concerns about cost were offset by his realization that we would not be spending much on travel and that the new landscaping, garden, and accessible outdoor space would be something that our whole family could enjoy. The added accessibility was particularly appealing to Ken at the time because the pain in his shoulders and arms was limiting his ability to use his wheelchair to get out to his favorite places in the yard. As I considered the size of the project, I prayed that the Lord would help me not let my imagination or enthusiasm for gardening outstrip His plans for me, my physical abilities, or our budget.

The new landscaping became a reality in the spring of 2000 and more than lived up to its promise. Its added benefits were yet another reason for much praise and thanksgiving to the Lord for His continuing blessings and provision.

Three years after this project was completed, I did retire from full-time work at Wheaton, although I continued to teach a popular seminar ("Psychology and Contemporary Mysticism") through the spring of 2007. My decision to retire completely in 2007 was motivated primarily by the fact that both Ken and I were struggling with some serious health issues.

My difficulties began rather abruptly in February of 2006. I started hearing a ringing sound in my right ear that rapidly grew much louder. I also felt pricking, pain, and numbness on the right side of my face and noticed hearing loss in my right ear. These symptoms would wax and wane in unpredictable ways, but over time they grew more intense. Medical tests ruled out a stroke or tumor, but neither our doctor nor the two specialists he recommended could identify the cause. After two more months without relief I tried to arrange an appointment with the neurology department at the Mayo Clinic. However, they rejected my application in spite of a recommendation from the doctor who had seen me there previously. He was puzzled because his patients had never been turned down before. I was confused and frustrated by the denial but eventually just concluded that the Mayo Clinic must not be where the Lord wanted me to go.

As an alternative, our family doctor recommended that I see a neurologist at the Loyola Medical Center in Chicago, so I made an appointment there. This doctor gave me a thorough examination, asked many questions, searched through my medical records, and entered all this data into the diagnostic software in his computer. However, after all of that, he was not able to make a diagnosis either. In obvious frustration, he ordered more tests, including a complete MRI of my spine! That confused me. Why order such an extensive test when my problem seemed so likely to be confined to my head?

I completed these additional tests. Later, the neurologist called me at home to tell me the results, ironically, right before we had planned to take two back-to-back weekend trips to visit with my family downstate. The tests had not shed any light on the symptoms he was trying to diagnose but did reveal a very small *tumor* in my left kidney. A radiologist had noticed it "by accident" while he was examining the MRI, while looking for possible abnormalities in my spine! The neurologist went on to say that he had sent this result to a urologist at Loyola and instructed me to make an appointment with him. But before that, he also wanted me to take two additional tests, one to determine whether the tumor was malignant and the other to see if it had spread!

Needless to say, we were blindsided by this news and deeply shaken by its possible implications. I immediately called Loyola and scheduled the tests and the appointment. As it turned out, I couldn't take these tests until after our first trip downstate, and I would get the results of the tests from the urologist late on the day we had planned to come back from our second trip.

At that point, we were uncertain about how to proceed. On the one hand, we were really looking forward to the trips as were other members of our immediate family who planned to travel with us. On the other, we were strongly tempted to cancel both trips because we didn't know how well we would function emotionally while struggling with the possibility that I might have cancer. We certainly didn't want to upset other family members unless that diagnosis was certain. Fortunately, and I believe by the Lord's prompting, we were reminded that we still did have a choice. We could either pray, choose to completely trust the Lord in this matter, and enjoy our visit, or cancel and likely waste much of that precious time being wracked by doubts and fears. Too often in the past, our first response to serious difficulty had been to become very emotional, imagining and then mulling over the worst possible outcomes. Only later would we come to our senses, yield the situation to the Lord, and experience His peace and direction. On this occasion, with His help, we were able to avoid most of that pain and useless flailing about.

We decided to stick with our plans and not even mention the possibility that I might have cancer to anyone until we knew for sure whether or not this was true. Our biggest challenge on this trip would be to continue trusting in the Lord's goodness and not let uncertainty and fear mar our visit. At first, actually doing this was very difficult. On the first trip, we sang along with many favorite hymns. These encouraged us, filling us with hope and gratitude for God's precious gift of eternal life. We would experience peace for a while, but then one or the other of us would succumb to fear and doubts. We had to *keep choosing* to trust the Lord each time. As we did so, God's peace and assurance began to prevail. Once I was with my family, I was able to push the threat almost entirely out of my mind, but for Ken, understandably, doing this was more difficult. The second trip downstate, a week later, was easier and more enjoyable. By that time, we had had more time to process my situation and gain more victory over our fears. This time the hymns elicited moments of deep joy, and God's peace was palpable.

Remarkably, that peace stayed with us after we returned and then went straight to the urologist's office to get the test results. He confirmed that I did have cancer, it hadn't spread, and the best and safest treatment would be to remove the left kidney. We could have panicked, but by that time, the events leading up to this office visit were forming a clear picture of God's intervention and guidance. We were also immediately reassured by the other things Dr. Perry had to say. Humans can live normally with just one kidney, and my right kidney was healthy. I would not need radiation or chemotherapy, because the cancer had been discovered at such an early stage. The chances that it would ever recur were only one in 100. Dr. Perry also informed us that he would be able to do the kidney removal laparoscopically (a fairly new procedure at the time), which would minimize the need to cut and further damage abdominal and back muscles that had been weakened by polio.

In spite of the bad news, Ken and I were so heartened by the obvious way the Lord was intervening in this situation that we were able to leave that appointment with hope and even joy! The very early discovery of the cancer had spared me from serious suffering and even an early death. And as Dr. Perry had predicted, the surgery and my recovery proceeded exceptionally well. In six weeks, I was basically back to normal.

Curiously, the facial and ear problems diminished and then disappeared shortly after the discovery of the tumor in my kidney, reappeared briefly in recovery right after the surgery, and then disappeared again for several months. When they appeared again, I also had a lot of pain in my gums around a lower back molar on the right side of my mouth. I went to my dentist for the tooth problem, and he discovered four severely impacted wisdom teeth. When an oral surgeon removed the teeth, the cause of the facial and ear symptoms also became apparent. One root of the wisdom tooth on the lower right side had wrapped itself around a branch of the facial nerve. As this root degenerated, it apparently irritated that portion of the facial nerve, and that was causing the symptoms! As added confirmation, the facial symptoms disappeared completely after my wisdom teeth were removed.

I was able to share this result with my neurologist in a final follow-up appointment. He looked very surprised and was obviously pleased that my problem had been solved, but he didn't say very much. However, I could see the gears spinning as he put the clues together and realized that this diagnosis made sense. I wouldn't be surprised if he eventually turned my very unlikely malady into a tough case study for his medical students to try to diagnose.

I believe that the unlikely chain of events in this situation provides a persuasive example of the Lord's intervention. My cancer was discovered early because I happened to be at Loyola for a strange set of neurological symptoms that no one could diagnose, leading my neurologist to order an unlikely and extravagant test. The radiologist who read this MRI "just happened" to notice that very tiny tumor in my kidney while looking for possible abnormalities in my spine. In this large teaching hospital, it was easy to transfer me directly to urology (which I later learned was one of the strongest departments at Loyola), to a doctor who did laparoscopic kidney removal routinely.

In addition, as I was to learn later, our situation was also covered by an amazing outpouring of prayer, from many places and people, including many who neither Ken nor I knew personally. A final confirmation of the Lord's hand in these events came several weeks later when our family doctor called me at home late one Friday afternoon. He had largely lost track of what was happening to me after I started treatment at Loyola. While sifting through a stack of reports from Loyola, he noticed that I had had my left kidney removed. He then traced back through the earlier events that had led to the discovery of the cancer. After briefly discussing this unlikely sequence of events with me, he told me straight out, "I do not know what you believe, but I am a Christian and I see evidence for God's hand and intervention in the way all this happened!" I did not know his beliefs before that time and was surprised and delighted by his bold statement of faith. It was a pleasure to tell him that I agreed completely and to rejoice with him in this clear example of God's guidance and provision.

While I was going through my difficulties in 2006, Ken was struggling with intensifying physical problems of his own. Because of increasing pain and weakness in his arms and shoulders, it was becoming difficult for him to push his manual wheelchair, even in the house, or to transfer to and from his wheelchair to the bed, the recliner, or elsewhere. So armed once again with many prayers for guidance and some good medical advice, we began acquiring equipment that would help us continue to function at home. This included, among other items, a special power chair, a well-designed hospital bed, and a power lift that ran on a track on our bedroom ceiling.

The power chair gave Ken a lot more freedom to get around inside the house, out in the yard, or at church, on shopping trips, etc. It was equipped with a detachable headrest so he could comfortably tilt it back at any angle. This enabled him to change his position frequently or even to nap right in the chair, decreasing the number of transfers he needed to make during the day.

The hospital bed also became an essential piece of equipment. Its controls allowed Ken to raise the head and foot of the bed independently, and that enabled him to shift to comfortable positions more easily during the night. The controller could also raise or lower the entire bed, which made transfers to and from the bed much easier. Ken could make the bed lower than his wheelchair when he wanted to transfer into the bed or higher than his chair when he wanted to transfer from the bed back into the wheelchair. That way he was always sliding "downhill" on his transfer board and did not have to use much arm strength to push himself along the board.

The last major piece of equipment we purchased was the power lift. That became necessary later when Ken began having difficulty making any transfers by himself. I knew from the advice of a nurse that I couldn't help Ken with a manual transfer lift. She warned me that these could be challenging for a person who was able bodied. However, on a visit to our local hospital, I saw a lift I knew I could use. It ran along a track mounted on the ceiling and was operated via a controller. I had Brian write down the name of the manufacturer. He was able to order it from the

Canadian manufacturer because he had his own remodeling business at the time. He and Niel reinforced the ceiling in our bedroom and then successfully installed the lift for us.

After I recovered from the kidney operation and we had the power chair and the hospital bed to use, our lives settled down to a "new normal" for quite a while. Although Ken's physical capabilities were diminished, we were still able to enjoy life and get out and do things together (even though doing so in two wheelchairs inevitably attracted more attention than we preferred). We went to church regularly, met with two couple's groups from the church, visited our grown children and their families, entertained at home, and went shopping for food together. I continued to garden and was able to do many things around the house.

That all began to change in early February of 2009 when I fell ill with a flu that caused heavy chest congestion. I recovered fairly quickly, but Ken caught the bug from me and within twenty-four hours developed a serious case of pneumonia. When I discovered that he was having trouble breathing, I immediately called 911, and he was rushed to our local hospital by ambulance. Neither a CPAP nor extra oxygen helped, so Ken was placed on a ventilator to keep him alive.

Ken remained in a drug-induced coma on the ventilator for days while his doctors administered various antibiotics to try to get the pneumonia under control. However, nothing seemed to work. After a few days, Ken's pulmonologist informed us that Ken's prognosis was not good. X-rays indicated that there had been extensive lung damage from the pneumonia, and the weaknesses in his diaphragm and chest muscles from polio were making his situation worse. He also cautioned us that Ken could not keep the ventilator tube in his throat indefinitely. If he didn't show improvement soon, we would be faced with a difficult choice. We could either have the tube removed and hope that Ken could begin to breathe with a CPAP machine and oxygen or allow the doctor to perform a tracheostomy and insert the ventilator tube there. However, doing this would also prevent Ken from swallowing food, so he would have to be fed via a stomach tube. In addition, he would not be able to talk and would probably be confined to bed. This arrangement would also mean that he could not stay at the hospital but would have to be transferred to a specialized long-term-care facility some distance from our home.

Years earlier, Ken and I had set up living wills, deciding that we didn't want our lives prolonged by artificial means if there was little or no chance for a meaningful recovery. I also knew that one of Ken's greatest fears was that he might become completely incapacitated and have to live the rest of his life in a long-term-care facility, in the care of strangers. So I understood in my mind what my choice had to be, but it was very difficult to imagine actually carrying it out. From the information we had at hand, removing the ventilator tube would likely lead to Ken's death in a matter of hours if not immediately.

Fortunately, I knew I didn't have to make this decision alone. Our family and fellow Christians were nearby for prayer and emotional support, and I asked our three grown children to help me make this choice. Faced with an impending deadline, we gathered at the hospital on a number of occasions to pray, search relevant scripture passages, consult with one of our pastors, Roger Crites, and to think through the options. After five days of this process, we each, independently, came to the same conclusion. No matter how difficult it would be to bear, we would ask that the ventilator tube be removed and entrust Ken's life to the Lord. Interestingly, Niel and I tended to believe Ken's doctors and were both pessimistic that Ken would recover. However, Brian, after deep and concerted prayer, had received what he believed to be a strong assurance from the Lord that Ken would live through this episode.

Surprisingly, on Ken's tenth day in ICU, right before the pulmonologist anticipated we would have to make our decision, Ken suddenly started needing less support from the ventilator. His improvement was rapid, and on the thirteenth day, the pulmonologist decided that this was the optimal day to act. Ken's chances of survival would probably start decreasing if he waited any longer. We hastily gathered at the hospital, prayed together, and waited anxiously for the outcome. To the utter astonishment of Ken's three doctors, who had predicted that it would take months for Ken to recover normal breathing if he did survive, when the ventilator tube was removed, he transitioned easily to breathing with oxygen alone. Moreover, within three days, *he was breathing normally without any oxygen at all!* All of us were delighted and were strongly convinced that we had just seen God's hand of intervention and healing. This simply wasn't Ken's time to die! Still, he had been seriously weakened by his bout with pneumonia, so he was sent to a rehabilitation hospital in Wheaton for further recovery.

After three days at Marianjoy, Ken's potassium levels rose to dangerous levels and he was sent back to Delnor Hospital by ambulance. Once again in the ICU, he developed serious chest pains from the potassium, and it appeared that he might die of a heart attack. He realized this and called each of our children to talk to him privately. He especially wanted to talk to Niel, who still had not fully accepted Jesus as his personal Lord and Savior. Niel told me later what Ken had said to him. "Niel, you need to turn your life over to Jesus. I want you to be with me in Heaven!" This had a powerful effect on Niel and was one of the factors that led him to do just that a few weeks later. Once more, we called for prayer for Ken, and yet again, God spared his life. Within a few more days, the cause of the potassium excess was uncovered and corrected, and Ken was sent back to Marianjoy. He made a rapid recovery there and finally came home on March 24, after seven harrowing weeks in hospitals.

After Ken came home, we had four wonderful months without any serious problems. We celebrated Easter together as a family, this time with a much deeper appreciation for its real meaning. We were privileged to celebrate Ken's seventy-ninth birthday with him in May. We celebrated a grandson's graduation from high school and, with Niel's help, even took a weekend trip to Barry so I could attend my fiftieth anniversary of graduating from high school. During this time, Ken also helped me learn how use the financial program on our computer and how to keep track of expenses and listed the things I would need to do if he were to die. Remarkably, he did this with great patience and complete peace. He also assured me that his former anxieties about death were now completely gone—he knew where he was going. During that time, I too had a very pervasive sense of assurance and peace.

On June 29, I came home after shopping for food and was shocked to see an ambulance and a fire truck in our driveway. Ken had called 911 himself. I knew he had a urinary tract infection but had no inkling that this could set off respiratory failure. I did not know until later that Ken had actually quit breathing and passed out in the ambulance before it left our driveway. Once again, Ken was quickly put back on the ventilator in ICU. However, this time he rallied quickly when the UTI was treated and once again successfully transitioned off the ventilator. This time he was home in eight days.

All seemed to be going fairly well after Ken came home, but this time our respite was only two weeks. Right after our hospital follow-up with our family doctor, Ken again became very short of breath, and he was back in ICU with respiratory failure. This time, he was not showing signs of improvement, and the pulmonologist informed us that Ken was dying and the only way to keep him alive was to do the tracheostomy, insert a stomach tube, etc. Once again, we committed Ken's life to the Lord and told the doctors we would not keep Ken on the ventilator. This time, we arranged for hospice care at home if he were to survive again.

When the ventilator was removed, against all apparent odds, Ken again cheated death. He continued to breathe, rallied, and did come home once more. On the second day home, he convinced the hospice aid to help him get into his power chair. We assumed that he just wanted to look around inside the house, but he wanted even more to go outside where he could travel on the brick walkway that circled our house so he could see the flower beds, the vegetable garden, and the large mature trees that framed our yard. We tucked a throw around his legs, and out he went. Ken was so overjoyed to be home once more, he cranked up the speed on his chair and literally went flying along the walkway, up and down the ramps to the deck, hospital gown partly flapping in the breeze. He even asked the aid to help him pick the tomatoes, one of the few jobs he could still help me do.

In the days that followed, Ken wanted to get dressed, get up in his chair, and continue with life as usual. We resumed our morning devotions together. Ken's mind was alert and sharp, and he was very much himself. In fact, he was doing so well that hospice discontinued continuous care. Just three days before his death, when our two sons, Brian and Niel, and Niel's wife, Mia, were visiting, we all participated in a remarkable conversation in our living room that none of us will ever forget. By this time, Mia had recommitted her own life to the Lord and Niel had made the same decision a few weeks after, persuaded by the extraordinary events that were taking place in Ken's and his own life at the time.

We listened to Niel speaking of his newly found faith, his changed perspectives, and his hunger to serve the Lord. We listened as Brian and Niel discussed their now common faith and listened as Ken, even in a weakened state, effectively addressed some of Niel's questions about the spiritual life. Ken was also able to hear both of his sons tell him that his consistent witness with his life was one of the main reasons they had become Christians. The air was charged with the Holy Spirit's presence, and we all just marveled at what was unfolding before us.

Yet even as we spoke, Ken was showing increasing signs of failing. His appetite had dropped sharply, his urine output was dwindling, and he was having bouts of uncontrollable sleepiness. We had planned to go to church on Sunday, but Ken didn't feel like getting up that morning. He slept a lot and very deeply that day, although he awakened in late afternoon when our daughter, Diane, and grandson, Douglas, stopped by for a visit. Afterward, as Diane and Douglas were leaving, Ken called Diane's name. When she turned to look back, Ken told her emphatically, "Diane, I will see you again!" Later that evening, she pondered that statement, because Ken did not say he would see her soon. Diane was occasionally haunted by some of the same fears of death that Ken had struggled with. After his death, she concluded, I think correctly, that this was his way of telling her to remember Christ's promise of eternal life and to remain strong for what was coming.

I had difficulty getting Ken comfortable and ready to sleep that Sunday night, so I called Niel and Mia and asked them to come and help. After we were finally able to get Ken settled, while we were discussing whether it might be a good idea for them to spend the night, I noticed that Ken was breathing very shallowly and pausing between breaths. As we watched, the pauses increased, and within fifteen minutes, he stopped breathing altogether. Without a trace of struggle or pain, Ken had slipped quietly into the arms of his Savior! While we were trying to come to grips with what had just occurred, we also caught a glimpse of just how powerful God's promises really are. Along with our grief and sadness, we also had peace and the strong assurance that Ken was now in Heaven. He had simply been called home before us, and one day we would be there with him, forever.

Chapter 14

Finishing Well

Not surprisingly, adjusting to Ken's absence in the weeks and months after his death was difficult for all of us. Still, there was much we could be thankful for. Ken had lived a long, meaningful, and productive life in spite of his serious physical disability. We were grateful for the strong biblical assurances that he was now in Heaven. And we were thankful for Ken's powerful example of faithfulness and courage. With the Lord's help, he had overcome many daunting obstacles and grown stronger in his faith and commitment to God with each victory. Our faith had also been greatly strengthened by the strong indications of God's intervention and timing in the events leading up to Ken's death.

Three times Ken had confounded his doctors and continued to breathe on his own when the ventilator tube was removed from his throat. Two times, our family and I had to act in faith, deciding to remove the ventilator at the risk of immediately ending Ken's life. And in spite of what had seemed inevitable to his doctors, Ken did not die in the hospital struggling for breath or in a long-term-care facility, as he had feared. He was able to return home, to finish equipping me so I could manage our affairs, and to interact in powerful and very meaningful ways with other family members. God's sovereignty over life and death were so evident so often during his last six months that none of us could seriously question God about anything that had happened. All we could do was to thank Him for so clearly revealing Himself and the truth of His promises.

Ken also left a legacy of faith that strongly impacted the lives of others and continues to do so through our family and others who knew him. It was his tenacious faith in God and the way he lived that helped persuade me to surrender my own life to Jesus. Ken's example also helped convince Diane, Brian, and Niel to make that same decision. By God's grace, all three are married to believers, and through their combined example, several of our grandchildren have also come to faith. Since Ken's death, others outside our immediate family have also accepted Jesus as their Savior through the witness of family members.

All of these things, plus the Lord's ongoing presence and comfort, helped me adjust to life without my husband. The grieving process was hard but not as difficult or disruptive as I had feared. Early in our marriage, I thought we might be fortunate to have twenty-five years together, so by the time we reached our forty-ninth anniversary, I felt that God had been incredibly generous. The six months that Ken was in and out of hospitals helped me anticipate and accept what was coming, so I didn't experience any deep shock or anger after Ken's death. I did go through significant bouts of grief, but these usually didn't last too long and became much less frequent and intense with time. Between episodes, I was able to sleep and function normally. It helped that our immediate family members lived fairly close by, so I could see them often.

To combat loneliness, I increased my involvement at First Baptist Church. During that time, Niel and Mia began attending a nearby Harvest Bible Chapel and asked me to come "check it out" to make sure it was biblically sound. I did and benefitted so much that I started attending there and at First Baptist on weekends.

In season, I also enjoyed working in my garden. In fact, it was shortly after working in the garden, roughly two years after Ken's passing, that I had my own close brush with death and yet another very strong confirmation of God's love and protection. It was a very warm July morning, and one of my granddaughters had been helping me set up a new watering system in the vegetable garden. We were just about finished when I noticed some dizziness and unusual sensations of pressure on my shoulders and neck. I assumed I was just getting too warm, so we finished what we were doing and moved inside.

I spent the rest of the day working alongside Rebecca in the air conditioning. When she left at about seven in the evening, I had a headache and a slight fever, felt somewhat ill, and noticed that my blood pressure was a little high. However, these symptoms didn't seem that unusual, and I was sure they would go away with a couple of Aspirin and a good night's sleep. I was definitely not alarmed by them.

Remarkably, in spite of my lack of conscious concern, a very strong, insistent thought kept recurring in my mind. I needed to prepare for an emergency ambulance ride that night! This seemed really strange. I did know what to do because I had called for an ambulance for Ken on several occasions. This thought was followed by what appeared to be clear, specific instructions. "Keep the portable phone where you can reach it." "Leave the door from the garage into the house unlocked." "Leave a note on the computer with your password." "Shower, but put on clean comfortable clothes instead of pajamas." "Leave your purse on the kitchen counter where it will be in plain sight." (My insurance cards were in the purse.)

At the time, this experience felt surreal. I obediently carried out each of these actions as they came to mind, all the while wondering if these were instructions from the Lord or just some strange harbinger of emotional instability. The likelihood of needing to call for an ambulance seemed very remote at the time. In fact, it seemed so unlikely that I didn't call Diane or Brian or Niel because I didn't want to alarm them for no reason and, frankly, because I was feeling pretty foolish about my actions. I had never done anything like this before. It was about ten o'clock when I pushed back in my recliner and fell asleep.

I awoke suddenly, around midnight, with sharp, heavy, relentless pain and pressure all across my chest. I knew immediately what was happening and breathed a quick prayer, "Lord, I don't know if this is my time to come home. If it is, Your will be done. If it is not, please help me do what I need to do." With that, I reached over, picked up the portable phone beside me, and dialed 911. The operator was calm, collected the necessary information, and I remembered to give her the number key that would open the garage door so she could relay it to the ambulance crew. The pain was intense, it was difficult to keep talking, and I realized that I didn't even have the strength to get out of the recliner by myself. However, I still had an incredible sense of peace! The ambulance crew came quickly, entered the house easily, and whisked me (and my purse) away, delivering me promptly to the emergency room at Delnor Hospital.

The ER doctor immediately ordered an electrocardiogram but didn't see any evidence of a heart attack on it and began looking for other causes for my chest pain. For reasons I can only attribute to God's provision, an excellent cardiologist was on hand at Delnor Hospital at that early morning hour, so the ER doctor conferred with him. The cardiologist did not see signs of a heart attack in the EKG either but was sure from my description of the pain, and the fact that nitroglycerine had relieved the pain in the ambulance, that this was a heart attack. He located an ultrasound machine that happened to be in the ER, dragged it into my cubicle, and quickly did an ultrasound himself. He looked startled and exclaimed that a large part of the left wall of my heart (part of the left ventricle) was not moving. He quickly asked my permission to do an angiogram and insert a stent if necessary. Somehow, he managed to scramble a team to carry out this operation in a matter of a few minutes between one and two o'clock in the morning.

Later, in recovery, I learned that Dr. VanDorpe had discovered a blockage in a major coronary artery dubbed the "widow maker." That artery was more than ninety percent blocked. Still later I learned that most patients do not survive with this type and degree of blockage. Time had clearly been of the essence. All the actions I had taken to prepare for the ambulance had been essential. It was crucial that the ambulance crew had moved rapidly and efficiently. It was critical that the cardiologist was immediately available to make a correct diagnosis. And it was vital that he had somehow found the help he needed so he could insert a stent in time to save my life.

Two other things were also remarkable about this event. In spite of the pain I experienced and the very real danger I was in, my heart had apparently suffered minimal damage. My heart enzyme levels remained low. I can only praise God for that! The other and most remarkable thing was that during this entire episode, the heart attack with its intense pain and my sudden recognition of my own helplessness, the ambulance trip, the high drama in the ER and the operating room and afterward in recovery, *I felt no fear!* These were all events that would have made me very fearful at earlier points in my life and would have made me very fearful on this occasion if I had been left to cope with this situation by myself. However, it was very clear from the start that I wasn't in this alone. The Lord's presence was very evident. I was experiencing the *"peace that passes all understanding"* (Philippians 4:7), which only the Lord can impart. Believe me when I say that there was no way I could have conjured up this peacefulness on my own!

As I noted in the introduction to this book, one of my reasons for writing this account was to share some of the amazing things Ken and I learned about the God who called us to Himself and then guided our journey through life. We learned a great deal *about* God and His purposes for our lives through church and Bible study. However, He allowed us to come to *know Him* through our times with Him in prayer, His amazing and timely answers to those prayers, His unfailing guidance, His lifelong provision for our needs and through compelling experiences of His presence and peace, right when these were most powerfully and obviously real.

The Bible teaches that God is the Creator of everything that exists—from matter and energy, all living things, to the entire universe. As the Creator, He is also infinitely powerful, wise, knowledgeable, and capable. Ken's and my own understanding and appreciation for these truths were powerfully reinforced by our training in the sciences. I know this may sound strange given the strident claims of some contemporary secularists who argue that modern evolutionary theories can explain our existence quite adequately without the need for a supernatural Creator.

Why this apparent contradiction? Here it important to recognize the differences between *scientific data*, that which scientists can actually see, measure, and predict using scientific methods, and their *interpretations* of that data. Scientists with very different worldviews can agree on actual physical data but can also disagree vigorously about what that data means or how to explain it. Although this might not be immediately apparent, scientists who deny that God is the Creator are also faced with some very formidable questions. For instance, if our universe, the sun and our earth, with all its varied forms of life, was not created by a being with vastly superior power and intelligence, how did this whole system ever come into being?

Those with a naturalistic bent rely on some variation of evolutionary theory to try to explain at least the origin of life. Their rationale is based on ideas from Charles Darwin's book, *Origin of the Species,* in which Darwin sought to explain how the great variety of current animal species alive on the earth today could have evolved, *by chance* and over millions of years, from a single, primitive, living cell, through the physical, unguided processes of mutation and natural selection. That book was published in 1859, and extensions of Darwin's theory became well entrenched in scientific thinking before scientists had the capability to actually see and truly appreciate the incredible complexity and precise operations of the many intricate molecular "machines" that enable each living cell to function.

At present, vastly improved microscopes and other powerful tools are revealing the mind-blowing complexity in even the simplest single cells alive today (bringing into question how even a "primitive" cell could have come into being by chance). There is now a growing appreciation that even the simplest cells are much more complex and intricate than anyone had ever imagined.

According to recent estimates, there are trillions of cells in the human body, and the great majority of these have DNA in their nuclei. Scientists have only recently begun to understand that this DNA actually functions like a very sophisticated *computer program* created by a human programmer! The probability that such detailed and clever instructions (or that the tiny and very sophisticated mechanisms within cells that use and were built according to these instructions) could come into being by chance, even over billions of years, is virtually zero. As one scientist, Stephen Meyer, has noted in his book, *Signature in the Cell*, it actually appears that God has placed His unmistakable signature on the DNA program in each cell so humans would eventually know for certain who created it, and also gave it that still mysterious property called "life"!

The Bible teaches that God is the Creator of *everything* and that His power, capability, knowledge, and wisdom are infinite— far above our ability to begin to appreciate. This is consistent with what is now known from scientific research related to our universe, our world, the living creatures and plants that inhabit the world, and human capabilities as well. From our training, both Ken and I could see that none of the cell-related phenomena mentioned above (or a multitude of other examples that could be cited) could possibly have come into being by chance. The mathematical probabilities of such are so infinitesimally small that they are simply not believable. On the contrary, God's creation, the precision with which it operates, its unbelievable complexity and intricate design literally shout our Creator's praises!

A second thing we learned, first hand, is that God cares deeply about the well-being of all people and is clearly involved in guiding the lives of those who come to Him through their faith in Jesus Christ. Neither of us could find any other way to explain why He enabled both of us to recover so much after polio, the astonishing way He worked through our circumstances to help each of us to attend college, to meet, to marry, to effectively provide and care for our children, to obtain advanced degrees, to manage with our own home, and on and on and on. Through all our lives, God has provided unfailingly for our present and future needs, often working behind the scenes to enable us to meet future challenges long before we even realized they were coming!

We also learned that God desires a close, personal relationship with each person and that He has a definite plan and purpose for each of us but will not force this relationship upon anyone. The way is open to all who are willing to acknowledge that He is God (and therefore has the authority to tell us how we should live), who will come to Him in the way He has provided (by faith in Jesus Christ), and begin (through the work of the Holy Spirit within us) to live and to grow to be more and more like Jesus.

As His followers, we need to submit our own wills to God's will and obey His instructions in the Bible, even though that goes against our strong natural preference to live our own way. His greater purpose for all who will come to Him through their faith in Jesus Christ is to deepen our relationship with Himself on this earth and, after death, to transform us completely with renewed minds and new imperishable bodies. In this new state, there will be no more sin, death, pain, or tears. And we have his promise that we will then live in unimaginable joy and fulfillment with our God, forever.

Because God purposes to begin our spiritual transformation in this life, believers encounter many struggles as well as many blessings. Like the perfect Father that he is, God uses discipline and rewards and punishments to bring about the needed changes. He provides many blessings, answers to prayer, and other wonderful things to enjoy. However, He also allows us to go through very difficult circumstances and applies serious discipline, as many times and in as many ways as necessary to help us learn to say "no" to sin and self-centered priorities, to trust and depend upon Him totally, and to grow stronger in our faith and love for Him and other people.

In our case, God used our physical disabilities, "impossible" challenges, recurrent struggles with sin and its consequences, and a variety of other tough situations to show us our own weaknesses, sinfulness, and lack of self-sufficiency. These taught us to rely more and more upon Him in prayer for our needs and upon the Holy Spirit, Bible study, and involvement with church and fellow believers for instruction and encouragement. As we learned to face new difficulties in this manner, God continued to answer our prayers in ways that met our needs and helped us to continue to grow in our faith and trust in Him. In this process, He also gradually revealed more of Himself, His will for our lives, and the depth of His love for us.

In retrospect, I think our physical disabilities simply exaggerated a condition that is common to everyone. When we try to live our lives entirely without God or His instructions for living in the Bible, we invariably run into trouble and disillusionment. It is only when we finally realize that we are not as smart, as strong, as virtuous, or as self-sufficient as we thought that we start searching for deeper meaning and purpose in life and become more willing to surrender our wills to the loving God who made us.

Because of the physical damage caused by polio, Ken and I were privileged to come to a clear understanding our own weaknesses and sinfulness early in our lives. And because we had to rely so much upon the Lord's help and provision, we also asked God for much more than we would have without those disabilities. But because our situation drove us to ask and trust God for so much, we were also privileged to see him respond by providing us with much, much more than we ever could have imagined or hoped for! (See Ephesians 3:20.) Through His continuing provisions and amazing answers to prayer, we came to understand just how real and awesome our God really is and how very much He loves all of those who will come to Him in complete surrender. These insights impacted both of us so deeply that we could even thank God for allowing polio to come into our lives, with all of the struggles and pain we faced because of it! (See James 1:2-4.)

One final point I need to stress is that neither Ken nor I received all the help and blessing that we did because we somehow earned or deserved it. These are simply gifts that God gives in different ways and different measure to *every* person who fully accepts Jesus Christ as his or her own personal Savior and Lord. If you would like to learn how you can begin your own relationship with God or deepen your understanding of this relationship, continue reading in the Appendix, "Developing a Personal Relationship with God," which follows this chapter.

If you have not yet made the choice to accept Jesus as your Lord and Savior, I urge you to do this without delay because the Bible warns that the consequences of not doing so or of rejecting God's offer are unimaginably horrible. Moreover, God's offer of relationship and eternal life is only open for a limited time. We no longer have the opportunity to choose that option after we die or after God brings final judgment upon the earth. Biblical prophecy and current events suggest that this judgment may be coming soon.

Developing a Personal Relationship with God

When considering a possible friendship with a new acquaintance, we usually try to learn as much as we can about that person before proceeding very far. This is also a logical first step when considering a relationship with God. The best place to learn more about Him is in the Bible, God's own words of instruction and encouragement for us.

According to the Bible, God has some of the same characteristics He created in human beings. Among these, He is a personal being capable of thought, language, making choices, and engaging in personal relationships, etc. However, God is also profoundly different from humans in many important ways. He is a spiritual being, uncreated and eternal, with no end and no beginning. His power, wisdom, knowledge, and other capabilities are unlimited. He exists outside the boundaries of time and is able to see the past, present, and future at will. He is also omnipresent, not confined to one place at a time but present everywhere. And He is omniscient, knowing everything, including all of our thoughts, actions, and motives. God is the Creator (and sustainer) of everything: the spiritual realm that He inhabits, the entire physical universe, and every living creature and person within it. His glory, majesty, and holiness exceed our ability to even imagine.

In the Bible, God is also described as loving (having strong affection and devotion toward those He loves), good (consistently thinking and acting in our long-term best interests), righteous (always acting in accord with His own perfect moral standards), and just (absolutely fair, rewarding what is good, and punishing what is evil by these same perfect standards). God does get angry and He does express his wrath, but unlike human beings, He always does so with perfect justice and righteousness.

The significance of our God-given abilities to form relationships

Meeting with friends, celebrating in family gatherings, rejoicing at the birth of a new baby, or enjoying the day-to-day companionship of a loving spouse are just a few of the gratifying interactions with other people that God has created us to be able to enjoy. In fact, engaging in interdependent relationships is an essential aspect of our lives, from infancy (e.g., a baby's complete dependence upon parents) to old age (when sons and daughters may be called upon to return the favor). In addition, our satisfaction with our lives is strongly correlated with the quality and depth of our relationships.

Curiously, because we are born with the capabilities and the need to engage in significant relationships, we tend to take the skills and abilities that make these relationships possible very much for granted. We do not usually appreciate just how complex and sophisticated they are or why God would go to such lengths to build them into us.

To illustrate, one very important capability that we depend upon in relationships is our ability communicate well with one another, through spoken or written words, facial expressions, tone and loudness of voice, posture, etc. Equally important is the ability of a listener to take in and rapidly process all the incoming verbal and nonverbal information in a conversation: recognizing words, remembering their meaning, comprehending what is being said, analyzing what it means, why the speaker said it, and how best to reply, all with split-second timing. Our ability to respond appropriately to other people is also learned, gradually, through our interactions with parents, siblings, and friends over the twenty-plus years that it takes to reach maturity. Ideally, these interactions will have also taught us correct values, obedience, respect for others, sharing, how to give and receive love, and much, much more.

Two other significant components of relationships are our ability to act independently of others and to choose between different courses of action. Choice plays a particularly critical role. For example, in an existing relationship between two people, both parties have already *chosen* to spend time together because of mutual attraction and benefit. Yet both have to *continue to make that same choice* for the relationship to last. If either party becomes dissatisfied, he or she can also choose to modify or end the relationship at will.

Of necessity, this summary of just a few of the skills that enable us to form relationships is very brief and incomplete. However, it should serve to demonstrate that these capabilities are very important to God. So what, we might ask, was His ultimate purpose for creating us this way? According to the Bible, God not only intends for believers (his adopted children) to enjoy loving relationships with one another, but also, as their heavenly Father, *desires a personal relationship with each of them!* In fact, much of the transformation believers experience here on earth is to help prepare them for a profound and eternal relationship with God in Heaven.

In our most cherished relationships here on earth, it is our knowledge that the other person's acts of kindness and consideration toward us are done voluntarily, primarily out of genuine love and concern for our well-being and not because they feel coerced or fearful or have some self-serving motive. Ideally, human relationships should be based upon genuine respect and mutual, unselfish love for one another. In the same way, God wants relationships with humans who choose to believe in Him, who want a relationship with Him, and who are willing to submit to His better plan for their lives to obtain it.

But herein lies a potential problem. How does God, who is so vastly superior and more powerful than we are, insure that we have a valid choice—accepting or rejecting His offer of relationship because that is what we want to do, not because we believe that is what we have to do in order to survive? If we were to catch even a glimpse of who God really is before we could make that choice or before we had learned of His love and amazing plan for our lives, that information could destroy our ability to choose. Likely, we would simply become so overwhelmed and fearful in His presence that we would quickly comply with anything He asked. We would be too afraid not to.

God's intention to give us a genuine choice in our relationship with Him may help explain why He so strongly veils His actual presence from us while we live upon this earth. The universe, the world we live in, and even our own bodies and being offer very strong *physical* evidence that there is an intelligent Creator. However, our lack of direct sensory evidence (actually seeing or hearing Him, as we would another person) also creates some uncertainty about His existence. This uncertainty effects people differently. It allows those who do not want a relationship with God to infer that God probably does not exist and, therefore, neither do His standards for living nor the consequences of ignoring them. That being the case, they feel free to justify and pursue any lifestyle or worldview they prefer.

By way of contrast, this same extended period of uncertainty allows those who will become believers to enter into a voluntary relationship with God. They must first choose to believe that God is real, then choose to carry out His requirements for relationship (i.e., accept Jesus Christ as their personal Savior), and finally, choose to begin to live the way God commands. In most cases, the time interval between making these choices and physical death gives believers numerous opportunities to experience God's guidance, encouragement, answered prayers, and love first hand while they are still on this earth. This evidence, in turn, strengthens their belief that God is real and that He really does love them as the Bible states.

Obstacles that can block a right relationship with God

The major obstacles that can block or hinder a personal relationship with God are His requirements for that relationship and human sin. God expects His followers to yield their wills to His and to live according to the rules and guidelines He has spelled out in the Bible. These requirements call for increasing obedience, self-discipline, and unselfishness on our part. By way of contrast, our strong natural bent is to control our own lives, satisfy our desires, and live as we please, even if that violates God's laws, dishonors Him, or brings harm to others or ourselves. Our acts of disobedience and/or disregard for God's laws are called *sins*.

According to chapters 2 and 3 of Genesis in the Bible, the first members of the human race lived in a paradise God created for them and enjoyed a close relationship with God, walking with Him in the garden and speaking with Him face to face. He gave them one simple command, which they could obey or disobey, warning them that if they disobeyed, they would die. When they chose to disobey, their relationship with God was broken, their lives were drastically changed, and they eventually died, as God had stated. We have inherited the same willful, sinful nature and disobey God's commands repeatedly. Consequently we also live with much pain and brokenness in ourselves, our families, our communities, and our world.

To summarize, we sin because that is now part of our nature ("me first"), because we want to control our own lives, and because we want to be free to engage in things God might prohibit. A fourth reason is that we fail to understand that God put His laws and standards in place for our own benefit. If we were all to live by them, we could live with others and in relationship with God in the best and most rewarding way possible. In His laws, God is simply asking that we accept Him as God, worship, love, and obey Him, and act with the same consistent, selfless love toward other people that He extends to us.

God gave the ten commandments (and other laws) to show us how He expects us to live. These are to worship God and God alone, not to worship false gods (idols), not to dishonor His name, to engage in regular communal worship, to honor one's father and mother, and not to murder, commit adultery, steal, give false testimony, or covet (e.g., desire for oneself what belongs to someone else). (See Deuteronomy 5:7-21.) Jesus was once asked which of these commandments was the greatest. He answered by summarizing God's general intent in all of them: *"'Love the Lord your God with all your heart and with all your soul and with all your mind.' This is the first and greatest commandment. And the second is like it: 'Love your neighbor as yourself.' All the Law and the Prophets hang on these two commandments"* (Matthew 22:36-40).

How does God respond to our sin? The short answer is that He hates it. Furthermore, His perfect righteousness and justice demand severe punishment for it. Therefore, sin brings two major consequences. First, the relationship that God intended for us to have with Him is broken. *"But your iniquities have separated you from your God; your sins have hidden his face from you, so that he will not hear"* (Isaiah 59:2). Second, we also face physical death, the separation of our spirits from our physical bodies. *"For all have sinned and fall short of the glory of God...the wages of sin is death"* (Romans 3:23, 6:23). Without God's further intervention, this dismal condition would continue indefinitely.

God's solution for our problem: "Jesus in our place"

Fortunately, God is not only righteous and just but also merciful, loving, and forgiving. Therefore, He did provide a way for those who would believe in Him to be saved. Because God is absolutely righteous and just, He could not simply ignore our sins. Yet neither can we pay the penalty attached to them (permanent death and separation from God) and yet be resurrected and remain in relationship with Him. God resolved this paradox by sending Jesus Christ, God the Son, to pay off our huge sin debt for us!

At the right moment in God's timetable of human history, Jesus (fully God and fully human) was born on earth and grew into manhood. He verified His divine nature with many miracles. For example, He demonstrated His power over nature by turning water into wine, walking on water, shriveling a fig tree with a word, and even stopping a violent storm at sea instantly with a simple command to "be still." He healed every kind of human injury or illness completely, instantaneously, and permanently. He even restored life to people who had died.

Jesus also began to teach the people around Him about the purpose of His coming. God was now providing a fail-safe way for anyone who really wanted to have their sin debt paid in full and to be reconciled with God to have that capability. In brief, God's solution for our problem has been called, "Jesus in our place." This can be somewhat difficult to comprehend, so before I continue my explanation, I would like to share a story that I once heard at church that helped me understand this provision better.

Once there was a ruler who was deeply concerned about the number of thefts that were occurring in his small country. In a desperate attempt to reduce these crimes, he finally decreed that any citizen found guilty of stealing should be beaten publically with many blows. In the course of time, his own aging mother was caught stealing. The ruler then faced a heart-wrenching dilemma. His mother was old and frail, and if she were beaten as prescribed, he was sure she would die. So what could he do? He loved his mother deeply and did not want to see her suffer or die, but he couldn't arbitrarily change his law

215

or try to make her an exception and still maintain justice. Justice needed to be carried out.

On the day of her punishment, as his mother knelt down to receive the beating, the ruler arose from his place of honor, strode out to his mother, leaned over, shielding her body with his own and ordered that the beating commence. He took his mother's punishment in her place, substituting his own body for hers, paying the price for her sin with his own suffering. By this selfless act, the penalty he had set in place was paid, and his mother was spared from horrible suffering and death. She felt great remorse for the pain and injury her selfishness had caused her son. She begged for and received his forgiveness, and their relationship was restored.

In our situation, Jesus Christ voluntarily took the punishment we deserve for our sins in our place. On the appointed morning, He bore the cumulative punishment for all the sins of every person, throughout human history, who would ever be reconciled to God. As predicted by the prophet Isaiah (about 700 years before it actually took place), this was accomplished when Jesus was tortured, crucified, and died on a Roman cross (see Isaiah 53). Death could not defeat the very one through whom life was created (John 1:1-3, 10-13), and in three days, Jesus arose from the grave with a resurrected body and with His primary mission accomplished. Jesus then remained on earth forty additional days, teaching His disciples and appearing to many other followers on different occasions. (Once He appeared to a group of more than 500. See 1 Corinthians 15:5-6.) On the fortieth day, while His disciples were watching, Jesus ascended into Heaven (see Acts 1:9-11).

After Jesus ascended, God didn't just leave the early believers alone to try to fend for themselves. He sent a powerful helper and teacher, the Holy Spirit, to live within each one, giving them the power, understanding, and other capabilities they would need to live and serve as God intended. The Holy Spirit still performs the same functions today, living within and helping each person who receives Jesus Christ as his or her personal Savior.

Without Jesus, all of us are under the sentence of death and eternal separation from God because of our sins. However, Jesus' sacrifice on our behalf gives us the opportunity to be released from this sentence, to live an abundant and meaningful life with God on earth, and after death, to dwell in full relationship with Him forever. God has also provided for the restoration of our bodies. At death, our spirit separates from our body. The spirits of believers go to dwell with God in Heaven, and the spirits of nonbelievers depart to a region of darkness and punishment separated from God to await final judgment (see John 5:24-30). Yet at God's appointed time, all the dead will be united with new bodies that are designed to last forever. Believers will be resurrected first, eventually living with God on a new earth where there will be no more sin, sorrow, death, or suffering—only joy, peace, love, and a complete realization of all that God originally intended for His creation to be. At a later time, nonbelievers will also be resurrected to receive what they have chosen—a life completely separated from God and from every good thing that He created humans to enjoy. According to the Bible, their final destination is in the lake of fire, in Hell.

What do we need to do to be reconciled to God and receive eternal life?

As a first step, ask yourself a few basic questions. Do you believe that there is a good, all-powerful God who wants a personal relationship with you and has a wonderful plan for your life? Do you agree with the biblical teaching that you are a sinner and have repeatedly disobeyed God's rules for living? Are you sorry for these sins and understand that living this way is wrong and is an offense to God? Do you believe that Jesus is the Son of God and that His payment for your sins on the cross can cancel your debt and allow you to be reconciled to God? Would you be willing (with the help of the Holy Spirit) to stop sinning and learn to live as God wants you to live? When you can honestly say "yes" to these questions, take the following steps:

1. Pray to God (speak to Him just like you would speak to another person) and tell Him that you really want a right relationship with Him but know that you are not worthy or capable of entering into this relationship on your own. Ask Him to help you.

2. Genuinely repent of your sins. Name the sins you are aware of and tell God that you are sorry for these and any other sins and ask for His forgiveness for them. Also tell Him that you intend (with the help of the Holy Spirit) to stop sinning and start living the way He wants you to live.

3. Affirm that you do believe that Jesus is God's Son, that He suffered and died on the cross to pay for your sins and triumphed over death and that He alone has the power to save you.

4. Continuing in prayer, receive Jesus Christ as your personal Savior. That is, invite Jesus to come into your life and to take control of your life through the presence and work of the Holy Spirit.

By praying through these steps, remember that you are making a deliberate choice and completing a transaction with God. If you have done this sincerely, several important changes take effect immediately:

1. God forgives you for all past sins, clearing the way for a meaningful relationship with Him. See Colossians 1:13-14, *"For he [God] has rescued us from the dominion of darkness and brought us into the kingdom of the Son he loves, in*

whom we have redemption, the forgiveness of sins. " Also see 1 John 1:9, *"If we confess our sins, he is faithful and just to forgive us our sins and to cleanse us from all unrighteousness."* (This verse also applies to sins we commit and confess after having received Jesus as our Savior.)

2. When you received Jesus, you were born into God's family through the supernatural work of the Holy Spirit who indwells every believer. See John 1:12, *"Yet to all who received him [Jesus], to those who believed in his name, he gave the right to become children of God."* As believers, we can consider and pray to God as our "Father" because when He saves us, He also adopts us as His own children (see Romans 8:12-17).

3. You received eternal life and the promise of a new body at the resurrection of believers. Remember these promises Jesus made: *"I tell you the truth, whoever hears my word and believes him who sent me has eternal life and will not be condemned; he has crossed over from death to life"* (John 5:24). *"He who has the Son has life; he who does not have the Son of God does not have life. I write these things to you who believe in the name of the Son of God so that you may know that you have eternal life"* (1 John 5:12-13). Read 1 Corinthians 15:35-56 to learn more about the resurrection of believers and our new bodies.

Next steps

Pray to God and read in the Bible at least daily, asking for guidance to help you live and begin to grow in your Christian life. Obtain a reliable translation of the Bible that is accurate and easy to read. I recommend the English Standard Version of the Bible (ESV) or the New International Version (NIV). You might want to start with an

ESV or NIV *Study* Bible, which includes many footnotes, maps, etc. that can help you better understand and apply what you are reading. If you are unfamiliar with the Bible, a good place to start reading is in the book of John, in the New Testament (located in the latter fourth of the Bible). John was one of Jesus' twelve disciples and gives an eyewitness account of Jesus' ministry, miracles, and purpose for coming to earth. The books of Matthew, Mark, and Luke also give accounts of Jesus' life and teaching. The Holy Spirit within you can also aid your understanding.

God didn't mean for us to try to live the Christian life alone, so if possible, you need to find a solid church (one that believes that the entire Bible is true) and interact with other believers to learn the essentials of the faith and continue to grow. Exercise caution here because there are currently many pastors and churches that are promoting false teachings. For instance, if they deny that Jesus was fully God as well as fully human or reject the idea that faith in Jesus is the only way to be saved from God's judgment or teach that we can be saved by our own good works, apart from faith in Jesus, their teachings are false. If you are sincerely trusting in God and praying regularly for His guidance, you will sense (and the Holy Spirit will confirm) that this is or is not the place you should be.

Finally, may God be with you, strengthen you, and bless you as you begin your own incredible (and challenging) journey to personal transformation, to a deep and abiding relationship with God, and to eternal life in a paradise we can scarcely even imagine. I look forward to meeting you there!